A Clinician's Guide to Cannabinoid Science

T0177342

Cannabinoid Science by Steven James tackles the issues surrounding the use of cannabinoids with a refreshingly objective tone that threads the needle between advocacy and opposition. Presented in a readable scientific voice, this book explores the history, the specific compounds, the mechanism of action and the distinct therapeutic targets of cannabinoids in a concise yet comprehensive style. Particularly useful are the bullet points at the beginning of each chapter summarizing chapter composition and the numerous references documenting the content. Nowhere else will the reader find the breadth of coverage of cannabinoids under one cover, nor is there any better source for the facts. This book is a must read both for clinicians wanting information about cannabinoids for their patients taking them as well as for patients themselves who want access to the best science available.

Dr Stephen M. Stahl, University of California at San Diego, San Diego, California

In this thoroughly researched, scholarly book, Dr James has drawn on his extensive experience interpreting clinical trials and his skill as a clinician to present a cohesive account of cannabinoid science. This is a valuable resource for anyone wishing to understand the clinical implications of this evolving field.

Dr Wallace Mendelson, expert in psychiatry and sleep medicine

A Clinician's Guide to Cannabinoid Science

Steven James
Clinical Assistant Professor of Psychiatry, University of California, San Diego

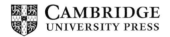
CAMBRIDGE
UNIVERSITY PRESS

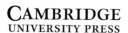

University Printing House, Cambridge CB2 8BS, United Kingdom

One Liberty Plaza, 20th Floor, New York, NY 10006, USA

477 Williamstown Road, Port Melbourne, VIC 3207, Australia

314–321, 3rd Floor, Plot 3, Splendor Forum, Jasola District Centre, New Delhi – 110025, India

79 Anson Road, #06–04/06, Singapore 079906

Cambridge University Press is part of the University of Cambridge.

It furthers the University's mission by disseminating knowledge in the pursuit of education, learning, and research at the highest international levels of excellence.

www.cambridge.org
Information on this title: www.cambridge.org/9781108730754
DOI: 10.1017/9781108583336

First published 2021

Printed in the United Kingdom by TJ Books Limited, Padstow Cornwall

A catalogue record for this publication is available from the British Library.

Library of Congress Cataloging-in-Publication Data
Names: James, Steven (Professor of psychiatry), author.
Title: A clinician's guide to cannabinoid science / Steven James, Clinical Assistant Professor of Psychiatry, University of California, San Diego.
Description: Cambridge, United Kingdom ; New York, NY : Cambridge University Press, 2021. | Includes bibliographical references and index.
Identifiers: LCCN 2020026272 (print) | LCCN 2020026273 (ebook) | ISBN 9781108730754 (paperback) | ISBN 9781108583336 (ebook)
Subjects: LCSH: Cannabinoids. | Cannabinoids – Therapeutic use.
Classification: LCC RM666.C266 J35 2021 (print) | LCC RM666.C266 (ebook) | DDC 615.7/827–dc23
LC record available at https://lccn.loc.gov/2020026272
LC ebook record available at https://lccn.loc.gov/2020026273

ISBN 978-1-108-73075-4 Paperback

....

For Lisa *Thank you for your patience over the many long hours. I am sure you are ready for a long vacation!*

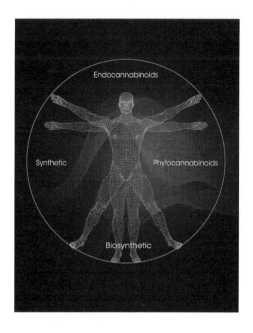

Contents

Preface

As to diseases make a habit of two things – to help, or at least, to do no harm.

Hippocrates, Of the Epidemics

When I decided to write "*The Clinicians Guide to Cannabinoid Science,*" I was unsure how this book would end. Perhaps that is the usual situation when a work of fiction is created by an author, but this seemed highly irregular in a book about science. Science is, after all, about data and facts. Over the course of my lifetime I have written, edited or read thousands of scientific papers and, although there were surprises, generally I could predict how the paper would end.

At the start of my career, I was immersed in the details of running clinical trials to develop better treatments for the care of my patients. Soon I became aware of how rapidly science progresses and the necessity for lifelong learning for myself and both the patient and the healthcare professional.

Originally, I had little interest in or awareness about marijuana and cannabis. As public interest and acceptance of cannabis grew, patients and colleagues would ask me questions that I could not answer. I had formed opinions, but they were based less on my limited knowledge about the science of cannabinoids and more on my biases. Probably the same is true for many of my colleagues in the healthcare professions and the general public.

Between 1999 and 2017 approximately 25,000 articles were published in the peer-reviewed medical journals, yet many textbooks used by clinicians as references to patient care included little or none of this information. Parallel to this flood of scientific knowledge on cannabinoids were the social and cultural movements to remove the prohibition of use and improved access. California was the first state in 1995 to allow the use of marijuana for medical conditions and the majority of states, Canada, many countries including most in the EU, Latin America, Australia and New Zealand have followed. Now, over a quarter of a century later, the trend continues with several countries and US states also legalizing recreational use.

I wrote this book because I could see daily the growing chasm between science and public opinion on cannabinoids. There is an opportunity to capture the moment and discover new treatments for devastating, hard-to-treat diseases but only if we are informed about the science. Hopefully this book will contribute to the scientific knowledge of clinicians and allow patients and society to be better informed.

When I decided to write this book, I chose to be the sole author. This proved to be a great challenge to me as I soon learned that cannabinoids touch nearly every aspect of human health. The endocannabinoid system is not an isolated system of interest to a few researchers but an immense network that regulates many physiological functions necessary to health.

I could not have written this book without the assistance of cherished colleagues who advised and corrected me when my knowledge was incomplete or wrong. My support staff were dedicated professionals and insured things were done well and on time even when I preferred to pause and reflect on what I had newly learned.

To Stephen Stahl, MD, PhD, my teacher, colleague and friend for nearly 40 years, thank you for your vision and support to have this book written. Wallace Mendelson, MD, another teacher and friend of also nearly 40 years, provided me guidance and inspiration to write this book. Without his encouragement this book would never have been attempted. Cristina Damatarca, MD, another long-term gifted colleague and friend, helped me identify the important safety issues we find ourselves confronting today with the parallel paths pursued by medical marijuana and discovery of new medicines from the pharmaceutical and biotech industries. Myles Jaffe, PhD, another long-term and cherished colleague, advised me on both the science and reminded me always focus on the truth. His comments were so insightful that after our discussions I would usually return to my writing with multiple revisions to every chapter. Renata Kisa, MD, a highly experienced dermatologists and medical educator, patiently explained to me the fascinating science of the skin. Greg DeLorenzo, MD, a prominent expert in rheumatology and superb physician, is also a friend that with his depth of knowledge and gift of communication helped me write the most difficult of chapters in immunology. I also wish to recognize and thank Robert Johnson, PhD, a young neuroscientist with knowledge and wisdom beyond his years. Robert helped me immensely to understand the role of cannabinoids and pain.

I also wish to express my deepest gratitude to Rose Freedland for her beautiful and inspiring illustrations for the book cover and chapters. I only hope the words I have written come close to describing what Rose has created. Alissa Williams provided the transcription of my hard-to-understand dictations and I hope the long chemical names and medical words were not too much of a burden. And a special thanks to Anya Gorban, a gifted artist that with eye to detail helped immensely in the final weeks of preparation for this book.

Finally, a special acknowledgment to the incredibly professional and capable team at Cambridge University Press. Catherine Barnes and Jessica Papworth have been marvelous!

An Introduction to the Botany and History of Cannabinoids

Chapter

1

Botany, the eldest daughter of medicine.
Johann Hermann Baas, Outlines of the History of Medicine and the Medical Profession

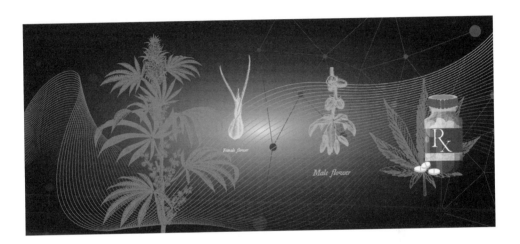

- Approximately one-fourth of all current prescription medicines are formulations that are either substances or derivatives of molecules from botanical sources.
- *Cannabis sativa,* also known as "marijuana," has been used for thousands of years. In 1964 Δ^9-tetrahydrocannabinol (THC) was first isolated and identified as the psychoactive constituent in the plant.
- In the late 1980s the first cannabinoid receptor that bound THC was discovered in the brain. Molecules referred to as endocannabinoids that bind to the cannabinoid receptors and are produced within the body were subsequently identified.
- Two types of cannabinoid receptors have been identified and are named CB_1 and CB_2. Cannabinoid receptors are G protein-coupled receptors widely distributed within the central and peripheral nervous system and multiple regions of the body.
- Phytocannabinoids are three-ring structures synthesized by the cannabis plant. Endocannabinoids are bioactive fatty acids derived from arachidonic acid in the body. Both groups bind to cannabinoid receptors.

Introduction

Plants have been a plentiful source of useful drugs and remedies throughout human history. In the early nineteenth century Friedrich Sertürner isolated morphine from the opium plant. By 1827, morphine was marketed by Merck in Germany and the origins of the modern pharmaceutical industry began. Over the remainder of the nineteenth century further advances in organic chemistry led to identification of other drugs from plant material. Examples of important medicines developed from plants included quinine from the bark of the cinchona tree for the treatment of malaria and salicylic acid from the willow tree that eventually led to the development of aspirin (Anderson, 2005). Today, the World Health Organization estimates that over 100 plant species are the source of approved pharmaceutical products and thousands of other plants are used for medical and recreational applications (Potter, 2014).

Progress in the identification of the constituents of cannabis (also known as marijuana) lagged behind the advances in plant chemistry. Although the cannabis plant has been used for fiber, as a medication, as a source of nutrition and as an element of religious ceremonies for over 4000 years, the constituents of the plant were extremely difficult to chemically separate because they were highly lipophilic, water-insoluble and frequently gelatinous. Isolating the substance that induced the psychoactive effect of cannabis was especially resistant to exploration (Iversen, 2008). Only in the 1930s was the structure of cannabinol (CBN) partially isolated by the British chemist Robert Cahn and work by Alexander Todd and Roger Adams in the 1940s in Britain and the United States came close to identifying cannabidiol (CBD) (Iversen, 2008). Finally, in 1964 Raphael Mechoulam and Yehiel Gaoni at Hebrew University separated $(-)\Delta^9$-tetrahydrocannabinol (also known as THC), a three-ring, 21-carbon terpenophenolic structure, from cannabis and demonstrated that the molecule was responsible for the psychoactive effects (Gaoni and Mechoulam, 1964). From this discovery followed 25 years of research that identified multiple naturally occurring cannabinoids from plants, referred to as phytocannabinoids and new compounds synthesized from chemical manipulation of the phytocannabinoid structure. The cannabinoids that were newly identified from cannabis were found to be extremely lipophilic and it was assumed that the action of THC likely occurred through nonspecific interactions within the neuron membrane (Iversen, 2008). The observation that THC activity was stereospecific (Mechoulam *et al.*, 1988) led to the search for specific targets that cannabinoids were likely to bind. In the mid-1980s Allyn Howlett at St. Louis University discovered the cannabinoid receptor 1 (CB_1) in the rat brain (Howlett, Qualy and Khachatrian, 1986; Devane *et al.*, 1988).

Obviously, a receptor in the brain is present to bind to an endogenous substance and not to specifically bind to a plant molecule and a search for an endogenous ligand began. A similar search had occurred earlier in the 1970s after the discovery of opiate receptors in the brain. That search ultimately led to the discovery of endogenously produced endorphins functioning within a previously unknown complex system of opiate receptors in the brain (Iversen, 2008).

Similar to the discoveries with opiates earlier, within a few years of the identification of the CB_1 receptor, the endogenous cannabinoid, N-arachidonoylethanolamide (anandamide; AEA), an ethanolamine of arachidonic acid, was discovered in pig brain using radiolabeled ligands by Mechoulam and Devane (Devane *et al.*, 1992). Later, a second endogenous cannabinoid, 2-arachidonoylglycerol (2-AG), an arachidonate ester of glycerol, was identified in canine intestines by the same investigators and in rat brain by Sugiura and colleagues (Sugiura *et al.*, 1995). Both AEA and 2-AG, referred to as endocannabinoids since they are synthesized within the body, bind to the cannabinoid receptor. However, the affinities for the cannabinoid receptors and the chemical structure of endocannabinoids differ significantly from the familiar three-ring structures of phytocannabinoids.

This discovery of the CB_1 and the binding of AEA and 2-AG was quickly followed by the identification of a second cannabinoid receptor (CB_2), initially located on white blood cells and spleen suggesting a role for cannabinoids in immune function and protection from attack and tissue repair (Munro, Thomas and Abu-Shaar, 1993). Although it was originally believed that the CB_2 was only a peripheral receptor, subsequent work found that CB_2 is also present in microglial cells in the brain.

It is possible that more cannabinoid receptors may be found in the future. GPR55 is a G protein-coupled receptor that binds THC and endocannabinoids (Derocq *et al.*, 1998; Ryberg *et al.*, 2007). CBD acts as an antagonist on this receptor and the CB_1 inverse antagonist rimonabant acts as an agonist at this site (Pertwee *et al.*, 2005). TRPV1 is another candidate and is a postsynaptic receptor that binds AEA in addition to activation by capsaicin. Both AEA and capsaicin bind to the same site within the cell and appear to mediate pain in sensory neurons (Starowicz and Przewlocka, 2012).

Brief History of Cannabis

The first historical record describing cannabis occurs in ancient Chinese literature dating from 2727 BC and the Chinese Emperor Shen Nung. Considered the "father of Chinese medicine," Shen Nung described hundreds of drugs from plants, animals and minerals in the Pen Ts'ao, believed to be the first pharmacopeia in history. The Emperor recommended in his work the use of hemp elixir to treat a wide range of ailments including gout and malaria. Although the original text no longer exists, the oldest surviving text of the Pen Ts'ao is found in the first century AD and refers to cannabis as "Ma," which is the Chinese word for chaos. We can only conjecture if the meaning of Ma and chaos was intended to describe the medicinal and psychoactive effects of cannabis. There is little doubt, however, that the Chinese regarded cannabis as a valuable medicine (Abel, 1980).

Probably as a result of invasion and migration from central Asia, cannabis arrived later to the subcontinent of India. Although the medicinal uses were also recognized, the Indian culture embraced cannabis as an important social and religious element. Legend states that Prince Siddhartha, later named Buddha, survived for six years exclusively on a diet of hemp seed in his quest for enlightenment. Later in Buddhism, cannabis was reserved for the priests and upper classes. Cannabis eventually became stratified into three classes: bhang, ganga and charas (known in other regions as hashish) and the use of cannabis became even more embedded into Indian culture (Booth, 2004).

Further awareness of cannabis extended beyond India into Persia, Syria and Greece. By 600 BC hemp was brought to the Middle East carried by the Indo-Aryan migration and was used both as a fiber and a medicine. In Syria cannabis was referred to as "qunubu" or the "drug for sadness" (Booth, 2004). The Greeks and Romans were certainly aware of cannabis as hemp and this played an important role in Greco-Roman society. Dioscorides, a Roman physician trained in the arts of Greek and Oriental medicine served in the Roman army during the first century AD and wrote *De Materia Medica* describing the medical uses of cannabis. *De Materia Medica* would remain among the most influential pharmacopeias in Western medicine for the next 1700 years (Abel, 1980; Booth, 2004).

In the Muslim era, there was little agreement if cannabis was an intoxicant or a medicine. In a culture where alcohol was prohibited, cannabis presented daunting religious questions. One resolution was to severely punish any recreational use of the plant while in other instances it could be used by physicians to administer treatment (Iversen, 2008).

Other uses were also found in the Muslim world. Hemp was used as a source of paper and later exported to Europe where it remained a medium of writing and printing until the introduction of wood pulp in the mid-nineteenth century (Abel, 1980; Booth, 2004)

The first reference to the term "hashish" is found in Egypt during the twelfth century AD and probably derives from the Arabic word for dried foliage. Hashish contains dried leaves and flowers along with the highly potent resin that was consumed originally by eating and not by the more common method today of smoking. The concept of burning dried plants to activate drug release in smoking was unknown until the sixteenth century with the importation of tobacco from the new world. Thus, according to legend popularized by the publication of Marco Polo's *"The Travels of Marco Polo"* in the twelfth century, another possible origin of the word hashish was from "assassins" that described the violent followers of an old man in the mountains (Booth, 2004).

Several trends converged in the nineteenth century and contributed to the growing awareness of the medicinal and psychoactive properties of cannabis in Western Europe. In 1839 William Brooke O'Shaughnessy, an Irish physician and professor of chemistry working for the British East India Company in Calcutta, presented the first medical paper on cannabis and hashish in western medicine to medical societies in India. In this paper he described his observations over seven years of the therapeutic effect of cannabis and hashish in the treatment of seizures, pain, fever and malaria and other conditions. O'Shaughnessy returned to London in 1842 where he published *The Bengal Dispensatory, and Companion to the Pharmacopoeia* that introduced to the British medical societies cannabis and other herbs used in India. He also provided hashish to a London pharmacist to make a medical extract with alcohol that was patented and sold as an analgesic. It was this extract that eventually found its way to North America as Tilden's Extract. So impactful were these activities that Queen Victoria is reported to have used cannabis for premenstrual pain (Booth, 2004).

O'Shaughnessy had a brilliant and open mind that saw the therapeutic possibilities of cannabis although he is better remembered in history for other work. He is credited with the first use of intravenous fluids for rehydration while a young physician recently out of training. Later, while in India, he was appointed Director-General of Telegraphs and built the first telegraph network in India. For this achievement he was knighted in 1856 (Booth, 2004).

Other events also contributed to the growing awareness that cannabis was more than a source of fiber. In 1796 Napoleon occupied Egypt with the design to disrupt British trade to the Middle East and India. Although he accomplished this goal of interfering with commerce, overall the mission was not a success. On August 1–3, 1798 the British navy under the command of Admiral Horatio Nelson defeated the French fleet at the Battle of the Nile. This effectively quarantined the French army of 35,000 men in Egypt and prevented supplies from France reaching them while the British blockaded the ports. It was during this time as the French were building fortifications to defend their occupation that the Rosetta Stone was discovered in July 1799 by Pierre-François Bouchard, an officer and engineer in the French army. Stranded in a Moslem country without alcohol, the French soldiers became acquainted with hashish much to the dismay of Napoleon. On September 2, 1801 the Capitulation of Alexandria was signed and the French army surrendered and were transported along with their supplies of hashish back to France by the British navy. The Rosetta Stone became the property of Britain and was shipped back to London and has been on continuous display in the British Museum since 1802 (Iversen, 2008).

Jacques-Joseph Moreau, a French psychiatrist, also contributed to this raising awareness about cannabis and hashish after studying about medical practices in India and China for several years. Returning to France in the 1830s, Moreau was the first to conduct clinical trials on psychiatric patients and described the effect of cannabis and hashish on the central nervous system (CNS). Moreau concluded that hashish could mimic mental illness but recognized that this action might also hold clues to potential treatment. From these observations the discipline of psychopharmacology arose (Booth, 2004).

Description of the Cannabis Plant

Cannabis is believed by many to have originated in central Asia or in the great river valleys of eastern China. Cannabis is an annual plant propagated by wind, widely distributed in temperate and tropical zones, and reported to grow at altitudes up to 8000 feet. The plant prefers direct sunlight, requires little water, germinates within six days and can reach maturity within five months. Because of its versatility, it is estimated that cannabis can grow in over two-thirds of the landmass of the globe (Booth, 2004).

In 1753 Carolus Linnaeus, the Swedish "father of botany," was aware of cannabis as hemp and its importance in rope and sail manufacture and named the plant "*Cannabis sativa*." Linnaeus chose the word "cannabis" from the Greek "kannabis" for hemp and "sativa" from the Latin word for cultivated. The evolutionary biologist Jean-Baptiste Lamarck in 1783 proposed a second species of the cannabis plant with the name "*Cannabis indica*" for a smaller, denser plant that grows in India. Lamarck believed that there were important distinctions between the two plants and noted that *C. sativa* possessed more fiber-like qualities and *C. indica* had more behavioral effects. Finally, in 1924 Janischewski, a Russian botanist, introduced a third species of cannabis named *Cannabis ruderalis*. *C. ruderalis* is found along the banks of the Volga River and in Siberia (Abel, 1980; Booth, 2004).

The appearance and geographic distribution of *C. sativa* and *C. indica* differ significantly. *C. sativa* is the more widespread of the two with the height of up to 15 feet. In contrast, *C. indica* can grow up to 4 feet in height and has dense branching and foliage (Booth, 2004).

Despite these differences in appearance and properties, controversy remains over classifying cannabis as several species (polytypic), or as one species (monotypic). Central to this argument is the belief that the observed differences may reflect the robust adaptability of the cannabis plant to different climates and soil. This view is based on the observation that seeds from *C. sativa*, when planted in regions where *C. indica* thrive, will over several generations display many of the characteristics of *C. indica*. In addition, the various types of cannabis can easily be interbred, cuttings can be cloned, and hybrids established resulting in myriad versions of the plant (Booth, 2004; Iversen, 2008).

The male plant produces pollen in the anther within a prominent flower while the smaller female flower after pollination produces seeds in the perianth.

The stem of the plant can be up to 5 cm in diameter and is covered with stiff fine hairs. When harvested and dried, the stem serves as the primary source of hemp and contains less than 0.3% tetrahydrocannabinol (THC). The distribution of THC varies in the plant with less than 1% THC in the leaves closer to the ground with increasing content up to 2–3% at the apex of the plant. Unpollinated female flowers do not produce seeds and contain higher THC concentrations up to 20%. When pollinated, seeds are produced and the concentration of THC in the flower is reduced since seeds do not contain cannabinoids. Thus, in the cultivation of cannabis for THC, male plants are usually removed from the growth area and only unpollinated female plants remain (Potter, 2014).

Both male and female plants produce a yellow colored resin containing high concentrations of THC in glandular structures at the base of the fine hairs. The resin is quite thick and sticky. Glandular secretions adhere to the male anthers and female perianths within the flowers increasing their cannabinoid content. In addition, female plants are prolific producers of resin compared with males. The purpose of the resin is unknown but may provide a natural protection for the plants against sunlight and heat as increased ambient temperature increases resin secretion. Others have speculated that the resin provides both a protective barrier and an impairing intoxicant that discourages insects and other pests (Potter, 2014).

Cannabis has a complex sexual physiology and usually each plant is one of two sexes (defined as dioecious). However, less commonly, individual plants may bear both male and female flowers and are termed hermaphrodites. Unpollinated female flowers do not produce seeds and are the preferred plant for production of cannabinoids while monoecious plants are cultivated for hemp and paper production (Booth, 2004; Potter, 2014).

Perhaps cannabis is best known today for the psychoactive properties exhibited when consumed. The psychoactive effect occurs when the phytocannabinoid THC traverses the lipid blood–brain barrier from the circulating bloodstream. Since all phytocannabinoids are extremely lipophilic, THC and the other compounds from the plant enter the brain with the well-known intoxication in addition to other non-psychoactive effects. In the blood, THC is converted into 11-hydroxy-THC and absorbed into fatty tissue. After approximately 30 minutes, THC is distributed back into the bloodstream. The phytocannabinoids exhibit a characteristic C_{21} terpenophenolic structure and within the plant other compounds including flavonoids and terpenes are to be found. The number of known cannabinoids exceeds 110 today and it is possible that others are yet to be found (Iversen, 2008).

THC is classified into three types based upon the concentration of the cannabinoid. Marijuana usually refers to dried leaves, flowers and stems. The THC content is between 5% and 10% and marijuana is the primary source of recreational use in North America. Hashish is made from the resin and glandular trichomes in addition to the flower and leaves of the cannabis plant. The resin contains high concentrations of all the cannabinoids and THC often exceeds 20%. Typically, the female unpollinated flower contains the most trichomes and highest concentration of cannabinoids and is the predominate constituent of Hashish. In Europe, hashish is the preferred form of THC in recreational use. Hashish oil is another version and may have THC content up to 85%. Typically, in most countries where THC is legalized, the hashish oil remains prohibited (Iversen, 2008).

The Cannabinoid System: Receptors and Neurotransmitters

Cannabinoids are molecules that alter neurotransmitter release by binding to cannabinoid receptors in the body. Cannabinoid receptors belong to the superfamily of G protein-coupled receptors (GPCR), a ubiquitous, 7-transmembrane family of protein receptors involved in the transduction of extracellular molecular messaging to intracellular response. After cannabinoids bind to the cannabinoid receptor, $G_{i/o}$-transduced inhibition of the enzyme adenyl cyclase results and the synthesis of cyclic adenosine monophosphate (cAMP), the second messenger for the intracellular signal transduction, is reduced. Through this second messenger system, binding at the cannabinoid is coupled with the mitogen-activated protein kinases that influence diverse signaling pathways within the cell (Mechoulam *et al.*, 2014).

The reduction of cAMP by binding at the cannabinoid receptor results in inhibition of calcium influx into the cell and is likely important in the reduction in neurotransmitter release. Most neurotransmitters are stored in vesicles and other mechanisms are involved in release into the synaptic cleft. It is possible these alternative systems may also prove important in understanding how cannabinoids influence neurotransmission.

Although cannabinoids binding at the receptor reduce neurotransmitter release, the overall effect of activation or inhibition is determined by the neurotransmitter that is inhibited. For example, glutamate and gamma-aminobutyric acid (GABA) are major neurotransmitters in the CNS and CB_1 receptors are found on these neuronal membranes. Glutamate is a ubiquitous neurotransmitter known to be activating and involved in tissue damage. Inhibition of glutamate by activation of the CB_1 receptor would be expected to result in reduced activation and even neuroprotection. In contrast, CB_1 receptors are also prominent on GABA neurons. GABA is the primary inhibitory neurotransmitter in the CNS and inhibition of GABA would result in increased activation and anxiety. Other neurotransmitter systems including the noradrenergic and cholinergic systems that are key systems in neurological and psychiatric disease are also known to be influenced by activation of the CB_1 receptor (Nestler, Hyman and Malenka, 2001).

CB_1 receptors were originally found in brain and were initially believed to be limited to the CNS. Later work has found that CB_1 receptors are also present in lesser amounts within peripheral tissue including heart, liver, fat tissue, stomach, intestines and testes. Despite this wide distribution throughout the body, the highest concentrations of the CB_1 receptor are in the brain and they have the highest density of any GPCRs. In the brain, the CB_1 receptors are distributed in the basal ganglia, substantia nigra, globus pallidus, hippocampus and cerebellum with little presence in the brain stem. The receptor is found predominantly on the presynaptic neuron axon terminal and this is an ideal location to influence neurotransmitter activity. The inhibition of synaptic transmission is the most common effect of CB_1 agonist activity.

CB_1 receptors are also found in the peripheral nervous system and are involved in sensory neurons, postganglionic sympathetic neurons, and in the parasympathetic nervous system. Because of the density of CB_1 receptors in the brain and wide distribution in diffuse organs, it is likely that when cannabinoids bind to the receptor significant physiological functions are influenced.

In close proximity to the CB_1 binding site, an allosteric site is situated on the membrane and, when activated, influences the primary CB_1 site. This modulation of CB_1 activity caused by the nearby allosteric binding can have significant effects including reduction or termination of response to the cannabinoid. (Price *et al.*, 2005). In the absence of cannabinoid binding to the CB_1 site, molecules that bind to the allosteric site will have no effect on the response.

The presence of endogenous allosteric molecules thus allows enhancement or diminution of the response to the primary binding site.

Just as the CB_1 receptor was originally thought to be only in the CNS, the CB_2 receptor was believed to be a peripheral cannabinoid receptor and involved in the immune response against protein attack and injury. Later studies confirmed that the CB_2 receptor is also present in the CNS especially in microglial tissue. Although the CB_2 receptor number is substantially less when compared with the CB_1 receptor in the CNS, the wide distribution in the body including cardiovascular, reproductive, gastrointestinal, pulmonary and hepatic systems suggest a broader role for the CB_2 receptor. Pacher and Mechoulam (2011) have speculated about a broad protective role of the CB_2 receptor by writing, "Are there mechanisms through which our body lowers the damage caused by various types of neuronal as well as non-neuronal insults? The answer is, of course, positive. Through evolution numerous protective mechanisms have evolved to prevent and limit tissue injury. We believe that lipid signaling through CB_2 receptors is a part of such a protective machinery and CB_2 receptor stimulation leads mostly to sequences of activities of the protective nature."

Cannabinoids are a major constituent of the cannabis plant. In mammals, two endocannabinoids have been identified that bind with a higher affinity to the cannabinoid receptors and have significant differences from phytocannabinoids in their chemical structure. Phytocannabinoids as previously noted are three-ring structures while endocannabinoids are long-chain fatty acids. A third class of cannabinoids are synthetic molecules manufactured in a laboratory setting and consists of various chemical structures that also bind to the cannabinoid receptor. Synthetic cannabinoids consist of multiple chemical structures including the three-ring structures of phytocannabinoids, eicosanoids, aminoalkylindoles, quinolines and others.

The phytocannabinoids are grouped into 11 types of cannabinoids. THC is the best-known cannabinoid due to its psychoactive properties. CBD is the other major constituent of the phytocannabinoids and has no psychoactive properties. Other cannabinoid types include (-)-Δ^8-trans-tetrahydrocannabinol, cannabigerol (CBG), cannabichromene (CBC), cannabinodiol (CBND), cannabielsoin (CBE), cannabicyclol (CBL), cannabinol (CBN), cannabitriol (CBT) and miscellaneous cannabinoids (Iversen, 2008).

THC is a partial agonist at both CB_1 and CB_2 receptors. Compared with endocannabinoids, the THC has a lower receptor affinity.

CBD, although non-psychoactive, may have important physiological properties. Research suggests CBD may work as a negative allosteric modulator on the CB_1 and CB_2 receptors. CBD may eventually demonstrate important benefits in the treatment of diverse diseases including epilepsy, psychiatric and sleep disorders, pain and inflammation. CBD may also have antioxidant effects and potentially provide neuroprotective benefits in neurodegenerative diseases such as the dementias including Alzheimer's disease.

The endocannabinoids consist of AEA and 2-AG. AEA is a N-derivative and 2-AG an O-derivative long-chain fatty acid. Unlike neurotransmitters that are stored in vesicles and wait for release, endocannabinoids are synthesized on demand and released immediately into the synaptic cleft to bind on presynaptic receptors. AEA is synthesized by phospholipase D and 2-AG by another enzyme named diacylglycerol lipase (DAG) (Di Marzo, De Petrocellis and Bisogno, 2005).

Both endocannabinoids are rapidly removed by a membrane transport process and inactivated. AEA is transported through this mechanism across the postsynaptic membrane and rapidly degraded by intracellular fatty acid amide hydrolase (FAAH) to arachidonic acid and ethanolamine. In contrast, 2-AG is transported across the presynaptic membrane and enzymatically deactivated by the enzyme monoacylglycerol lipase (MAGL) (Dinh, Kathuria and Piomelli, 2004).

Similar to the situation with cannabinoid receptors, other endocannabinoids are likely to be discovered since other lipid molecules interact with the cannabinoid receptors or share some common metabolic pathways or targets.

Fatty acids are widely distributed throughout the body but have significant differences in the amount and distribution of the lipid and their degradative enzymes. Both AEA and 2-AG are derivatives of arachidonic acid which is a polyunsaturated fatty acid commonly found in cell membranes and is especially prominent in the brain. Arachidonic acid is known to be involved in cellular signaling and as an inflammatory intermediate and differences in the distribution of degradative enzymes may lead to different roles for the two endocannabinoids.

AEA has been found throughout the brain and peripheral tissue and can be present where the CB_1 receptor is highly concentrated or has limited distribution suggesting that the molecule may be important in other non-cannabinoid processes. AEA is a partial agonist at the CB_1 receptor and can act as a weak partial agonist/antagonist at the CB_2 site.

2-AG is more prominent than AEA and has been proposed as the primary endocannabinoid for the known cannabinoid receptors (Sugiura et al., 2002). Unlike AEA, 2-AG is a full agonist of both CB_1 and CB_2 receptors. Because of the differences in concentration and binding affinity to the cannabinoid receptors, it has been suggested that these two endocannabinoids have different roles to play within the cell (Maccarrone, Dainese and Oddi, 2010; Alger and Kim, 2011).

Other arachidonic acid derivatives are also known to act on cannabinoid receptors: 2-arachidonoyl glyceryl ether (noladin) (Hanus et al., 2001), virodhamine (Porter et al., 2002), and N-arachidonoyldopamine (NADA) (Huang et al., 2002).

The Pharmacokinetics of Phytocannabinoids

Although the cannabis plant contains multiple cannabinoids, terpenes and flavonoids, THC and CBD have been the most important and studied due to their prevalence and pharmacodynamic effects. Smoking is the most common route of administration although oral ingestion is a frequent option.

Smoking results in rapid absorption in the lungs and distribution of cannabinoids to the brain. The euphoriant effects from smoking cannabis are the result of the rapid uptake into the CNS of THC. As might be expected with smoking, there are large differences in dose-dependent individual choices of depth and length of inhalation. Peak plasma concentrations (C_{max}) of THC absorbed from the lungs occur within 6–10 minutes and peak concentrations are only slightly less from smoking when compared with intravenous administration. Bioavailability is defined as the percentage of unchanged drug that reaches the systemic circulation and is 25% of plasma concentrations by 10 minutes. Because smoking allows the user to "titrate" the dose, there is considerable variation in the mean concentrations after 15 and 30 minutes.

It is estimated that between 2 and 22 mg of THC must be administered to experience the psychoactive effects of THC. With a bioavailability of approximately 25%, this suggests that between 0.2 and 4.4 mg is the dose that must be smoked (Parker, 2017).

THC is highly fat-soluble and can also be ingested as a food or liquid. Under these conditions the absorption is considerably delayed and there is a reduced peak level in comparison with smoking. Time to peak value occurs after 2–6 hours (compared with less than 10 minutes by smoking) with bioavailability lower (6%) compared with smoking (25%) (Huestis, 2005).

THC is metabolized by the CYP 450 system to the equipotent 11-hydroxy-THC and the inactive 11-nor-9-carboxy-THC metabolites and glucuronide conjugates. Cytochromes 2C9, 2C19 and 3A4 are involved in the metabolism to the 11-hydroxy-THC and the plasma concentration of this metabolite is about 10% of THC after smoking and approximately equivalent after oral ingestion. As discussed earlier, more than 100 other metabolites have been identified from the metabolism of THC and there is no effect by gender (Huestis and Smith, 2014).

Within five days the majority of THC and its metabolites are cleared from the bloodstream and eliminated primarily in stool (65%) and urine (25%). Hydroxylated and carboxylated metabolites are the most common with the carboxylated glucuronide primary in urine and the 11-hydroxy-THC in stool.

THC is rapidly removed from the bloodstream due to its high lipophilicity and is absorbed in organs richly supplied by the vasculature including the heart, lungs, brain and liver. While the blood flow to fat tissue is more limited, THC is more slowly absorbed into adipose tissue but sequestered for a longer duration. For this reason, inactive THC metabolites may be detected in plasma for up to a month after conception although the intoxicant effects of THC have long subsided (Huestis and Smith, 2014).

Endocannabinoids structurally are much different from the phytocannabinoids and the synthesis, distribution and elimination differ dramatically from the phytocannabinoids just discussed. Endocannabinoids will be discussed in detail in Chapter 3.

Regulation of Cannabis in the Twentieth Century

In 1909 the USA and China convened the first opium conference to address the growing concerns regarding opium and other drugs of potential abuse. From this meeting, international restrictions were imposed on the exportation of opium, cocaine and cannabis.

Neither the USA nor China, however, were signatories of the international treaty signed at the Hague in 1912. Both countries were dissatisfied with simple restrictions on exportation agreed at the conference and advocated for prohibition of cannabis and opium cultivation and sale. Later in 1925, a second opium conference was held and sponsored by the League of Nations in Geneva. This time the participants agreed to the prohibition of cultivation and production of hashish. One exception to this was the Indian government which held the position that hashish represented an important social and religious role in the Indian culture and refused to accept this decision.

For the next 30 years this agreement was in force and survived the world war and the development of synthetic opiates by the pharmaceutical industry. However, by 1960 it was clear that the agreement needed to be updated to reflect the scientific advances in the pharmaceutical industry.

The International Single Convention on Narcotic Drugs was convened in 1961 with the objective of updating existing international agreements and providing flexibility to accommodate future scientific advances. An outcome of the conference was the establishment of a classification of potentially addictive drugs into five schedules. At the time, the cannabinoid responsible for the psychoactive effects had yet to be identified by Mechoulam and his group in Israel. Perhaps for this limited knowledge, the cannabis plant and all its substances and derivatives were classified in the most restrictive schedule along with opium and cocaine.

One objective of the convention was to establish a format that member nations could follow and develop their individual internal regulations consistent with international agreements. In 1969 the US Congress began consideration of the Controlled Substances Act to align US drug law to international agreements. President Nixon signed the act into law in 1970 and cannabis was classified as a Schedule I drug. With this designation, prohibition of use in humans became law with substantial penalties and access to cannabis for preclinical and clinical trials became severely limited. This designation was determined by Congress during the drafting of the bill and included provisions that future additions or deletions from scheduling would reside under the authority of the US Drug Enforcement Agency (DEA) in the Department of Justice and the US Food and Drug Administration (FDA) (Mead, 2014).

Shortly after the US passage of the Controlled Substances Act, the United Nations in 1971 held the UN Psychotropic Convention and recognized that THC was the psychoactive component of cannabis and would remain as a Schedule I drug. The other constituents in marijuana including non-psychoactive cannabinoids, terpenes and flavonoids would subsequently be placed in less restrictive schedules. Many countries have recognized this decision and revised their drug schedules to reflect this change. The USA and Canada, however, were exceptions to this trend and maintained all cannabis products in the most restrictive classification until very recently.

Bibliography

Abel, E. L. (1980) *Marijuana: The First Twelve Thousand Years*. New York: Plenum Press.

Alger, B. E. and Kin, J. (2011) 'Supply and demand for endocannabinoids', *Trends in Neurosciences*, 34, 304–315.

Anderson, S. (ed.) (2005) *Making Medicines: A Brief History of Pharmacy and Pharmaceuticals*. London: Pharmaceutical Press.

Booth, M. (2004) *Cannabis: A History*. New York: St. Martin's Press.

Derocq, J. M. *et al.* (1998) 'The endogenous cannabinoid anandamide is a lipid messenger activating cell growth via a cannabinoid receptor-independent pathway in hematopoietic cell lines', *FEBS Letters*, 425 (3), 419–425.

Devane, W. A. *et al.* (1988) 'Determination and characterization of a cannabinoid receptor in rat brain', *Molecular Pharmacology*, 34(5), 605–613.

Devane, W. A. *et al.* (1992) 'Isolation and structure of a brain constituent that binds to the cannabinoid receptor', *Science*, 258 (5090), 1946–1949.

Di Marzo, V., De Petrocellis, L. and Bisogno, T. (2005). 'The biosynthesis, fate and pharmacological properties of endocannabinoids', *Handbook of Experimental Pharmacology*, 168, 147–185. doi:10.1007/3-540-26573-2_5.

Dinh, T. P., Kathuria, S. and Piomelli, D. (2004) 'RNA interference suggests a primary role for monoacylglycerol lipase in the degradation of the endocannabinoid 2-arachidonoylglycerol', *Molecular Pharmacology*, 66(5), 1260–1264.

Gaoni, Y. and Mechoulam, R. (1964) 'Isolation, structure and partial synthesis of an active constituent of hashish', *Journal of the*

American Chemical Society, 86(8), 1646–1647.

Hanus, L. *et al.* (2001) '2-arachidonyl glyceryl ether, an endogenous agonist of the cannabinoid CB1 receptor', *Proceedings of the National Academy of Sciences of the United States of America*, 98, 3662–3665.

Howlett, A. C., Qualy, J. M. and Khachatrian, L. L. (1986) 'Involvement of Gi in the inhibition adenylate cyclase by cannabimimetic drugs', *Molecular Pharmacology*, 29(3), 307–313.

Huang, S. M. *et al.* (2002) 'An endogenous capsaicin-like substance with high potency at recombinant and native vanilloid VR1 receptors', *Proceedings of the National Academy of Sciences of the United States of America*, 99, 8400–8405.

Huestis, M. A. (2005). 'Pharmacokinetics and metabolism of the plant cannabinoids, delta9-tetrahydrocannabinol, cannabidiol and cannabinol', *Handbook of Experimental Pharmacology*, 168, 657–690.

Huestis, M. A. and Smith, M. L. (2014) 'Cannabinoid pharmacokinetics and disposition in alternative matrices', in R. G. Pertwee. (ed.), *Handbook of Cannabis*. Oxford: Oxford University Press. pp. 296–318.

Iversen, L. (2008). *The Science of Marijuana*. Oxford: Oxford University Press.

Maccarrone, M., Dainese, E. and Oddi, S. (2010) 'Intracellular trafficking of anandamide: new concepts for signaling', *Trends in Biochemical Sciences*, 35, 601–608.

Mead, A. P. (2014) 'International control of cannabis', in R. G. Pertwee (ed.), *Handbook of Cannabis*. Oxford: Oxford University Press. pp. 44–64.

Mechoulam, R. *et al.* (1988). 'Enantiomeric cannabinoids: stereospecificity of psychotropic activity', *Experientia*, 44(9), 762–764.

Mechoulam, R. *et al.* (2014). 'Early phytocannabinoid chemistry to endocannabinoids and beyond', *Nature Reviews Neuroscience*, 15(11), 757–764.

Munro, S., Thomas, K. L. and Abu-Shaar, M. (1993) 'Molecular characterization of the peripheral receptor for cannabinoids', *Nature*, 365(6441), 61–65.

Nestler, E. J., Hyman, S. E. and Malenka, R. C. (2001) *Molecular Neuropharmacology. A Foundation for Clinical Neuroscience.* New York: McGraw-Hill Company.

Pacher, P. and Mechoulam, R. (2011) 'Is lipid signaling through cannabinoid 2 receptors part of a protective system?', *Progress in Lipid Research*, 50, 193–211.

Parker, L. A. (2017) *Cannabinoids and the Brain.* Cambridge, MA: MIT Press. p. 29.

Pertwee, R. G. *et al.* (2005). 'Evidence that (-)-7-hydroxy-4-dimethylheptyl-cannabidiol activates a non-CB (1), non-CB (2), non-TRPV1 target in the mouse vas deferens', *Neuropharmacology*, 48(8), 1139–1146.

Porter, A. C. *et al.* (2002) 'Characterization of a novel endocannabinoid, virodhamine, with antagonist activity at the CB1 receptor', *Journal of Pharmacology and Experimental Therapeutics*, 301, 1020–1024.

Potter, D. J. (2014) 'Cannabis horticulture', in R. G. Pertwee (ed.), *Handbook of Cannabis*. Oxford: Oxford University Press. pp. 65–88.

Price, M. R. *et al.* (2005) 'Allosteric modulation of the cannabinoid CB1 receptor', *Molecular Pharmacology*, 68(5), 1484–1495. doi:10.1124/mol.105.016162.

Ryberg, E. *et al.* 2007. 'The orphan receptor GPR55 is a novel cannabinoid receptor', *British Journal of Pharmacology*, 152(7), 1092–1101.

Starowicz, K. and Przewlocka, B. (2012) 'Modulation of neuropathic pain related behavior by the spinal endocannabinoids/endovanilloid system', *Philosophical Transactions of the Royal Society of London. Series B Biological Sciences*, 367, 3286–3299.

Sugiura T. *et al.* (1995) 'Arachidonoylglycerol: a possible endogenous cannabinoid ligand in brain', *Biochemical and Biophysical Research Communications*, 215, 89–95.

Sugiura T. *et al.* (2002) 'Biosynthesis and degradation of anandamide and 2-arachidonoylglycerol and their possible significance', *Prostaglandins, Leukotrienes and Essential Fatty Acids*, 66, 173–192.

Δ⁹-Tetrahydrocannabinol (THC) and Cannabidiol (CBD)

Let us permit nature to have her way. She understands her business better than we do.

Michel de Montaigne, Essais

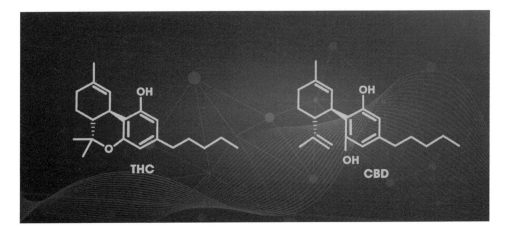

- Δ⁹-Tetrahydrocannabinol (THC) and cannabidiol (CBD) are 2 of over 100 phytocannabinoids produced by *Cannabis sativa* and are the most extensively studied of the botanical cannabinoids. In addition to phytocannabinoids, other biologically active molecules including terpenes and flavonoids are present in the cannabis plant and many have biological properties similar to the cannabinoids.
- THC is a *partial* agonist for both cannabinoid receptor 1 (CB₁) and cannabinoid receptor 2 (CB₂). The CB₁ receptor contains two binding sites referred to as the orthosteric site and allosteric site. Binding by THC to the orthosteric site on the CB₁ receptor produces the euphoriant effects of marijuana.
- CBD has little direct agonist activity for the CB₁ or CB₂ receptors. CBD binds to the CB₁ allosteric site and changes the conformational structure and binding affinities of the CB₁ orthosteric site.
- Binding of CBD to the CB₁ allosteric site has no physiological effect when agonism of the orthosteric site is absent. This may account for the blockade by CBD of some THC effects but the absence of CBD activity when THC is absent.
- Both THC and CBD bind to cannabinoid receptors and to a large number of non-cannabinoid receptors, transmitters and transport systems. These non-cannabinoid targets account for many of the effects associated with plant-based cannabinoids.

Cannabis sativa is known to contain over 100 phytocannabinoid compounds plus a mixture of other molecules including terpenes and flavonoids. Collectively, well over 500 different compounds are known to naturally occur in *C. sativa* and very likely many intriguing properties and potential uses of *C. sativa* still await discovery. Δ^9-Tetrahydrocannabinol (THC) and cannabidiol (CBD) are two of the most common cannabinoids present in the plant and considerable scientific attention has been devoted to these common, but very different, cannabinoids.

Δ^9-Tetrahydrocannabinol (THC)

THC is the primary psychoactive constituent of the cannabis plant and is best known for the "high" associated with marijuana. It is the most abundant phytocannabinoid present in *C. sativa* and was first isolated in 1964 at Hebrew University by Gaoni and Mechoulam (Gaoni and Mechoulam, 1964). Once isolated and the molecular structure identified, chemical synthesis quickly followed and the greater psychoactive potency of the (-) trans isomer compared with the (+) trans isomer was identified. This stereoselective property of a molecule extracted from a plant that could bind to a receptor in an animal was an unexpected discovery. This suggested that phytocannabinoids bind to these sites that had other specific functions and interact with unidentified ligands produced within the body. Within the next 25 years at least two cannabinoid receptors (CB_1 and CB_2) in the body were identified that were activated by the plant-based phytocannabinoids. Once these receptors were found, the discovery of the internal ligands later termed endocannabinoids followed along with their synthetic and degradative enzymes. The cannabinoid receptors, endocannabinoids and their enzymatic pathways are now referred to as the endocannabinoid system (ECS). Phytocannabinoids (including THC and CBD) are not part of the ECS but express many of their effects on the body through this system. Prior to the discovery of the ECS, a similar finding of opioid receptors in the body that bound opioid molecules originally derived from plants had led to the understanding of the endorphin system. Together, these two discoveries of the ECS and the endorphin system revealed surprising insights into the functions of the body that have yet to be fully understood.

Once the ECS had been described, it was recognized that THC was a partial agonist at both the CB_1 and CB_2 receptors rather than a full agonist. In some ways this should not be surprising since phytocannabinoids present a three-ring molecular structure that differs significantly from the naturally occurring endocannabinoids that are long-chain fatty acids. In addition, phytocannabinoids obviously evolved to serve a beneficial function for *C. sativa* and their activity with the ECS was likely coincidental. Perhaps the role of phytocannabinoids evolved as a protective system for the plants as these molecules are known to have toxic effects on insects and other threats to the cannabis plant. Although the function phytocannabinoids may serve for *C. sativa* may be open for conjecture, the perhaps more interesting question why the ECS evolved in vertebrates also deserves to be answered. In Chapter 3 endocannabinoids will be introduced and their role in maintaining homeostasis in human health discussed.

Later THC was found not only to have partial affinity for the CB_1 and CB_2 receptors but to have a broad range of interactions with non-cannabinoid receptors, transporter systems and enzymes found widely throughout the body. THC and its psychoactive effects as a partial agonist at CB_1 receptors has drawn great attention although the majority of the physiological effects of THC occurs outside the ECS.

When first discovered the CB_1 receptor was thought to be expressed only in the central nervous system (CNS). It is now recognized that CB_1 is present in other organs in addition to the CNS and includes the cardiovascular, pulmonary, gastrointestinal, skin, immune and ophthalmic systems Although this receptor is highly expressed within the CNS, the broad diversity in multiple organ systems suggests that the ECS serves an important function in the body. The additional activity of phytocannabinoids on non-cannabinoid receptors in the body only reinforces the findings that cannabinoids have many functions. Several of these actions and their potential benefits will be introduced later in Section 2.

Within the CNS, the CB_1 receptor is especially plentiful in several regions including the cortex, basal ganglia and cerebellum. A second area where CB_1 is abundant is the limbic lobe and hippocampus. The plentiful expression of CB_1 in these brain areas likely underlies how THC may modulate motor activity and emotional feeling respectively.

Early rodent studies firmly established this affinity of THC and the other cannabinoids for these areas of the brain. Subsequent preclinical animal studies revealed other consistent effects on the CNS including hypothermia, cataplexy and antinociception (Martin et al., 1991; Adams and Martin, 1996). These recurring results eventually became recognized as the "tetrad" effects of cannabinoids: namely locomotion, hypothermia, cataplexy and antinociception and follow-up work with THC in humans identified additional effects on motor control that included impairment of fine motor control (Greenberg et al., 1994). Other effects including appetite simulation, regulation of nausea and vomiting, analgesia and sleep have been associated with THC and are now well-accepted properties. Several of these findings have led to development of approved pharmaceutical products starting in the 1980s. These prescription drugs based initially on THC will be discussed further in Chapter 4.

As a partial agonist, the affinity of THC for the CB_1 and CB_2 receptors is relatively low compared with full agonists and is influenced by several factors. Obviously, receptor site availability and the amount of THC present are important. Many exogenous and endogenous compounds (including, but not limited to, endocannabinoids) can compete for access to the binding site. In addition, cannabinoid receptors can undergo a process referred to as dimerization where the receptor combines with itself or other types of receptors. This fusion of two receptors sometimes of different classes leads to conformational changes that can account for some of the complex outputs from the ECS. This will be further discussed in future chapters of this book.

Non-endocannabinoid Receptors

The cannabinoid receptors are the most abundant family of receptors within the CNS although activation of non-cannabinoid targets mediates numerous properties of THC. GPR55, originally classified as a putative third cannabinoid receptor, and GPR18 are both classified as orphan receptors. GPR55 is a prominent G protein-coupled receptor in the CNS and GPR18 is found peripherally in lymphocytes and THC is believed to have affinity for both. GPR55 plays a role in eating behaviors and has been associated with body weight, body mass index (BMI) and fat percentage (Moreno-Navarrete et al., 2012). Although there is some controversy whether THC has any meaningful interaction with GPR55, some studies support binding to GPR55 (Lauckner et al., 2008; Ryberg et al., 2009; Pertwee et al., 2010) while others have been unable to establish an effect. GPR18, in contrast, is more firmly established as a binding site for THC (McHugh et al., 2012; Penumarti and Abdel-Rahman,

2014). Both GPR55 and GPR18 have been associated with the modulation of pain and may provide a pathway for antinociceptive effects of THC.

Serotonin, also known as 5-HT, is synthetized mainly in neurons located in the raphe nucleus of the brain stem. From these neurons, an extensive network of axons projects to higher brain regions including the limbic system and cerebral cortex and cellular communication is modulated by THC. Robust antagonist effects at the 5-HT_{3A} receptor by THC are recognized as the likely mechanism where the well-established anti-nausea and anti-vomiting effects of THC are expressed (Pertwee et al., 2010). Dronabinol, the first synthetic cannabinoid approved as a pharmaceutical product in 1985, was initially approved for the indications of anti-nausea and antiemetic effects.

Glycine is another neurotransmitter located in the brain stem, hippocampus, spinal cord and retina. This amino acid is similar to another inhibitory neurotransmitter gamma-aminobutyric acid (GABA) and is generally found in cytosol but also stored in synaptic vesicles. The glycine receptor is a chloride-containing ionophore. Abnormalities of glycine are associated with severe neurological deficits in children with associated motor disease. THC potentiates glycine activity and this may be another mechanism for THC to play a role in reducing pain (Hejazi et al., 2006; Pertwee et al., 2010; Xiong et al., 2012).

Surprisingly, although there seems little doubt that THC reduces pain, there is no known interaction with the TRPV1 receptor. This receptor is located intracellularly in postsynaptic neurons found in the trigeminal ganglion and dorsal horn of the spine. When the receptor is activated by capsaicin (hot pepper), a reduction in pain occurs (Gregg et al., 2012). THC agonist activity is found, however, with other TRPV family receptors and this may be another mechanism through which THC contributes to pain relief. As a family of receptors, the TRPV receptors are associated with the perception of pain, pressure and temperature (De Petrocellis et al., 2012).

The opiate system is another area of intense interest. There is a well-established interaction between the cannabinoids and the opiate system. THC functions as an allosteric modulator at the δ and μ opioid receptors and it has been proposed that this effect may prevent opiates from binding to their natural sites (Kathmann et al., 2006). This displacement of opioids from the opioid receptors has led to speculation that cannabinoids may serve a beneficial role in the treatment of opioid abuse although this remains a controversial topic and will be the topic of further discussion in Chapters 5 and 6 of this book.

PPARγ receptors are found within the cell and are situated on the nuclear membrane. When activated, these receptors regulate transcription of genes associated with fatty acid storage and breakdown of glucose. Multiple ligands in addition to the phytocannabinoids have been reported to bind to nuclear PPARγ receptors. Some have speculated that affinity to these receptors mediate neuroprotective and anti-inflammatory properties and contribute to the analgesic properties of THC (O'Sullivan, 2007; Pistis and O'Sullivan, 2017).

Pharmacokinetics of THC

Unsurprisingly, inhalation of cannabis is the most common way THC is consumed. At approximately 200 °C THC becomes vaporized when smoked and the molecule is rapidly absorbed and detectible in plasma. THC is then metabolized primarily through the hepatic cytochrome isoenzyme CYP2C9 to 11-hydroxy-THC and by CYP3A4 to 8-β-hydroxy-THC. The psychoactive metabolite 11-hydroxy-THC is then converted by cytochrome P450 isoenzymes to 11-nor-9-carboxy-THC (Burstein, Rosenfeld and Wittstruck, 1972). Compared with THC, the metabolites all have a slower uptake and reduced peak levels. Only 15–50% of inhaled THC is absorbed with the remainder of the cannabinoid lost through sidestream smoke or broken down by pyrolysis (Brenneisen, 2007). The inactive 11-nor-9-carboxy-THC metabolite persists for several days in the blood and is the molecule usually detected in urine drug screens for cannabinoids.

Once absorbed in the lungs, THC is quickly distributed to highly vascularized organs including the brain. Because cannabinoids are extremely lipophilic, inhaled THC easily penetrates the blood–brain barrier and binds to multiple cannabinoid and non-cannabinoid targets previously reviewed within the CNS.

Experienced smokers appear able to carefully titrate the dosage of the inhaled drug, compared with novice users. Differences in the amount inhaled, duration of smoking, and the rapid passage to the brain enables the experienced user to carefully titrate the dosage sometimes up to twice the peak level compared with the inexperienced user for desired results. Peak levels of THC have been reported at 9 minutes with decline in levels to 60% by 15 minutes and 20% at 30 minutes (Huestis, 2007).

Oral consumption is an alternative route to administration but is more variable compared with inhalation. Typically, THC is dissolved in a lipophilic solution such as sesame oil or solid foods with high fat content. After it is ingested, THC is absorbed in the intestines after passing through the acidic environment of the stomach where it is partially degraded. Absorption is frequently erratic with peak levels achieved within 1–4 hours. Hepatic enzymes present a significant first pass effect with less than 10% of THC available for systemic distribution (Halldin et al., 1982). Because of the variability in absorption and delay in CNS effects, oral consumption is harder for the user to titrate and can lead to overingestion of the cannabinoid and adverse events. Other oral routes for THC include oromucosal sprays and liquid oral solutions of synthetic molecules. Several formulations using these oral routes are approved including in the United States, Canada and the European Union. In Chapter 4 these approved medications will be further reviewed. It is important to be aware that although inhaled THC is the most common route of administration, it is not approved for prescription use anywhere in the world.

Rectal administration is another uncommon route to administer THC and bypass the liver. There is limited information on the route of administration although the bioavailability appears to be increased compared with oral absorption. However, there is extreme variability in absorption between individuals limiting any benefit from this route.

The volume of distribution of THC is approximately 10 L/kg body weight with deposition in multiple body sites including adipose, liver, heart, lung, intestine and renal. THC and its metabolites are highly bound to circulating lipoproteins with less than 3% of free THC available (Brenneisen, 2007).

Plasma clearance is similar to hepatic blood flow and THC is rapidly eliminated from the circulation (Harvey and Mechoulam, 1990; Harvey, Samara and Mechoulam, 1991). After inhalation, peak values occur rapidly in plasma and can persist for up to 2 hours. After oral ingestion, peak values are delayed and can occur up to 4 hours. Although the psychoactive components are rapidly metabolized, the non-psychoactive metabolites undergo further hydroxylation or carboxylation and elimination can occur over several days (Halldin et al., 1982). For some metabolites, sequestration in adipose tissue may persist for several weeks (Agurell et al., 1986; Harvey, 1999). About one-third of THC and its metabolites are excreted in urine with the remainder in feces.

Drug–Drug Interactions of THC

As discussed earlier, THC is metabolized by the cytochrome P450 isoenzymes CYP2C9 and CYP3A4 (Yamaori *et al.*, 2010). Apparently studies in cytochrome P450 inhibition and induction by THC have found only limited potential for drug–drug interaction although, as will be discussed later in this chapter, this is in contrast to CBD (Stout and Cimino, 2014). THC also binds strongly to proteins although coadministration of other protein-binding drugs has not been reported as problematic.

Although concerns about drug–drug interactions appear fairly limited, synergism with other drugs could potentially result in problematic side effects. As an example, sedation and effects on the heart (such as tachycardia) are associated with THC and can be especially troublesome to manage and metabolism of theophylline may be enhanced (Grotenhermen, 2002).

It is well established that coadministration of CBD with THC may moderate the observed effects of THC. There is no pharmacokinetic effect that has been associated with coadministration of THC and CBD with no change in clearance, volume of distribution and half-life (Huestis, 2007).

Cannabidiol (CBD)

CBD was first extracted by Roger Adams at the University of Illinois and then chemically synthesized in 1942. The isolated CBD consisted of minor impurities and the complete purification and identification was not completed until over 20 years later. Although technical limitations presented barriers to purification of the molecule, the 1940s were also an era of prohibition of marijuana in the USA and this restriction likely inhibited the research into CBD and other cannabinoids.

The discovery of THC in 1964 by Raphael Mechoulam and his associates in Israel proved the tipping point in modern day research of the cannabinoids. THC was quickly identified as psychoactive and research quickly expanded to identify and learn about the multiple molecules including revisiting CBD within the cannabis plant.

As we discussed in Chapter 1, the cannabis plant contains over 100 different cannabinoids and derivatives plus numerous terpenes and phenolic compounds including flavonoids. THC, the most plentiful cannabinoid, and the 11-hydroxy metabolite remain the only psychoactive components found in cannabis. CBD, devoid of psychoactive properties, is the second most abundant phytocannabinoid in cannabis and has become the object of intense scientific inquiry due to its multiple effects. The absence of psychoactive effects is an obvious benefit and many of the actions of CBD appear to modulate or counter the effects of THC including changes in mental status. Other beneficial properties in the treatment of epilepsy and schizophrenia have also been identified and a purified extract of CBD has been approved for use in several rare epilepsies of childhood in the USA and EU. Other potential uses including psychiatric, neurodegenerative and autoimmune indications discussed in Section 2 of this book further broaden the interest in CBD.

CBD shares the three-ring structure of the other phytocannabinoids and differs only from THC as an open ring in one of the three structures. This small difference in structure, however, results in major differences in the three-dimensional molecular structure and results in significant differences in the interaction of CBD with the ECS. We have already discussed that the CB_1 receptor consists of two binding locations described as the orthosteric binding site and an adjacent allosteric site. CBD has little direct affinity for the orthosteric site that binds THC and other cannabinoid agonists but binds to the nearby allosteric site. This allosteric binding initiates conformational changes to the main orthosteric site and alters the affinity for CB_1 agonists such as THC in addition to the endocannabinoids N-arachidonoylethanolamide (anandamide; AEA) and 2-arachidonoylglycerol (2-AG). Thus, although CBD has little direct influence on the orthosteric site important for CB_1 receptor properties, major effects through modulation of the cannabinoid receptors occur.

Similar to THC, CBD also influences the ECS through multiple activities independent of the cannabinoid receptors. In the presence of CBD, the uptake of AEA from the synaptic cleft into the cell for breakdown is inhibited possibly through an effect on the membrane transport system. In addition, degradation of AEA once in the cell by the fatty acid amide hydrolase (FAAH) is also reduced by CBD. As a result, the presence of CBD indirectly increases endocannabinoids and results in greater availability of AEA to bind to presynaptic targets.

Non-endocannabinoid System Activities of CBD

The ECS is only one of many systems of cellular communication influenced by CBD. Similar to THC and the other phytocannabinoids CBD interacts with an expanded group of targets outside the ECS. These non-cannabinoid activities represent the majority of physiological effects of CBD. Numerous enzymatic systems, ion channels, and transporter systems offer plentiful opportunities for CBD in addition to the cannabinoid and non-cannabinoid receptors.

As previously discussed, GPR55 and the peripheral GPR18 are important targets of CBD. As discussed earlier in this chapter, GPR55 is sometimes referred to as the "third cannabinoid receptor" in part due to the structural homologies shared with the transmembrane domains of the cannabinoid receptors. In contrast to THC, CBD acts as an antagonist or inverse agonist to GPR55 and GPR18. Both endocannabinoids AEA and 2-AG also serve as agonists to these receptors in contrast to the actions of CBD (Brown, 2009).

CBD also binds to other non-cannabinoid receptors. Glycine, serotonin, cholinergic, opioid and peroxisome proliferator-activated receptors (PPARs) are only a few of the many sites of activity for CBD.

Cannabinoid interaction with glycine receptors, as discussed earlier, may play an important role in the reduction of chronic pain. In one rodent study, systemic and intrathecal injections of CBD significantly reduced inflammatory and neuropathic pain without developing tolerance to the analgesic effect (Xiong et al., 2012)

The adenosine receptor also is known to be a target of CBD. There are at least four different adenosine receptors and CBD may be involved through the A_1 receptor in the regulation of coronary blood flow and oxygen consumption in the myocardium (Gonca and Darıcı, 2015) and possibly in the forebrain where the receptor is involved in temperature regulation and sleep. CBD is also known to be a potent inhibitor of the inflammatory properties of neutrophils possibly through influence on the cellular uptake of adenosine. There is also evidence that CBD may demonstrate neuroprotector properties although this has yet to be conclusively proven (Sagredo et al., 2007, 2011).

Serotonin (5-HT) is another important target for CBD. Although found throughout the body including platelets and mast cells, within the brain serotonin-containing neurons are found in the pons and upper brain stem. There are at least eight different subtypes of serotonin receptors and CBD has been reported to bind as an agonist at the 5-HT_{1A} and 5-HT_{2A} receptors. In vitro studies comparing the properties at the two sites suggest that CBD has weaker affinity for the 5-HT_{2A} receptor and may be a partial agonist (Russo *et al.*, 2005).

There is some evidence in rodent studies that CBD may modulate μ and δ opioid receptors (Kathmann *et al.*, 2006) and nicotinic acetylcholine receptors in in vitro investigations (Mahgoub *et al.*, 2013).

In human cancer cell lines, CBD has been found to interact with the nuclear membrane PPARγ receptor and to inhibit tumor cell viability (Ramer *et al.*, 2013; Hinz and Ramer, 2019). As noted earlier, PPARγ receptors are influenced by endogenous substances that generally are lipids and further evidence remains to be obtained to understand the specific effect of CBD on this receptor.

Phytocannabinoids interact with multiple enzyme systems. CBD interacts with the cytochrome P450 system including inhibition of CYP2C9, CYP2D6 and CYP2C19 and some evidence for CYP3A4, CYP3A5 and CYP3A7 (Jiang *et al.*, 2011). Recent clinical studies of a relatively pure CBD (Epidiolex [cannabidiol]) in childhood epilepsy reported elevation in liver enzymes when coadministered with clobazam further confirming the effect of CBD on liver enzymes.

In a recent literature review, CBD was identified to have effects on 32 specific enzymes. In addition to the cytochrome P450 system, FAAH, important in the degradation of the endocannabinoid AEA, enzymes involved in redox reactions, cholesterol metabolism and apoptosis, phospholipases and others have also been identified. Overall, the authors estimated that 49% of molecular targets for CBD were enzymes with only 15% receptors that included CB_1 and CB_2 (Ibeas Bih *et al.*, 2015).

Pharmacokinetics of CBD

As interest grows in the breadth of activity and potential therapeutic value of CBD, understanding the pharmacokinetics of the cannabinoid will become evermore important. CBD is one of the most used herbals in the USA and Europe and determination of dose, maximum benefit and duration of effect will become critical to use it effectively and safely (Harvey and Mechoulam, 1990; Harvey, 1999). It is surprising that only very limited information is known about the pharmacokinetic and pharmacodynamic properties of these commercialized herbs sold as medicine to patients. This will be discussed further in the summary of this chapter and in Chapter 5 dealing with safety.

Ingestion of CBD, like THC and the other phytocannabinoids, occurs through different routes and each method has a unique and well-established pharmacokinetic profile. Consumption usually occurs through inhalation although intravenous (IV), sublingual, oral, transdermal and rectal routes have also been used. Differences in formulation also play an important role in pharmacokinetics of the cannabinoid.

In a recent literature review (Millar *et al.*, 2018), 24 peer-reviewed papers were identified after surveying the medical literature that reported CBD pharmacokinetics in humans. The majority of these reports evaluated CBD in combination with THC or cannabis. Despite the widespread use, CBD alone in humans was studied in only eight studies with one study of bioavailability in humans.

Although the IV route is rarely used, it is an important approach to understand the pharmacokinetics of CBD without the many confounding variables associated with cannabis consumption. An early IV study using deuterium-labeled CBD was published in 1986 and compared the IV administration of 20 mg CBD with inhalation of 19.2 mg of the phytocannabinoid. After IV administration, CBD peaked at 3 minutes with plasma levels of 686 ng/ml and after 1 hour the plasma CBD declined to 48 ng/ml. Bioavailability of the smoked CBD was reported at 31 +`13%. Plasma clearance was calculated at 960–1560 ml/min. The half-life was reported to be 24 hours (Ohlsson *et al.*, 1986).

CBD when delivered by inhalation is typically included in a combination of phytocannabinoids and terpenes and rapidly absorbed by the lungs and distributed to the brain. Inhalation is the most common means of delivery typically administered in cannabis and avoids the delay of the first pass effect of CBD to the brain. Through inhalation, the bioavailability has been reported to be as high as 31% (Grotenhermen, 2003) with peak levels within 10 minutes. Pyrolysis of CBD and sidestream smoke account for the remainder of the CBD inhaled. Similar results are found in studies using a vaporizer CBD and THC (Newmeyer *et al.*, 2016).

Oral delivery and absorption across the oral mucosa with drops or spray offers an alternative route to deliver CBD and shares the advantage of limiting the first pass effect of the liver. Compared with inhalation, however, this is a less efficient route of delivery with some CBD inevitably swallowed and metabolized by hepatic enzymes. Oromucosal delivery provides an alternative means of administration with rapid absorption resulting in peak plasma levels less than inhaled. The half-life of CBD after oromucosal spray varies from 1.4 to 4.2 hours.

Oral formulations of CBD including liquid, capsule and tablets, and edible cannabis-based foods are increasingly consumed. Absorption of CBD is extremely variable perhaps due to the high lipophilicity of the molecule. Bioavailability of orally consumed CBD is estimated to be 6% and is significantly lower compared with the other methods and obviously varies depending on the formulation and composition of the CBD consumed. (Hawksworth and McArdle, 2004). CBD is substantially metabolized by the hepatic microsome systems resulting in a significant first pass effect that further reduces plasma levels after absorption (Grotenhermen, 2003). Absorption from oral consumption may occur from 45 minutes up to several hours.

Formulations including oils, gels and creams have also become increasingly popular with CBD. Transdermal delivery of cannabinoids offers many potential benefits compared with oral administration including consistent plasma levels and less frequent dosing intervals. Similar to inhaled, transdermal also avoids the first pass effect of hepatic metabolism. For these reasons, CBD transdermal is of great interest and the permeability of the skin to CBD has been reported to be superior to topical application of THC. When applied in an ethanol solution as a tincture, CBD can achieve tissue concentrations 10-fold greater than THC (Stinchcomb *et al.*, 2004).

In a recent canine study, absorption of transdermal CBD delivery was compared with that of an oral-infused CBD and oral microencapsulated CBD oil beads. CBD plasma levels were obtained during acute and chronic administration. The oral-infused CBD resulted in the best availability of CBD, and the transdermal was the least effective (Bartner *et al.*, 2018).

After absorption into the body, CBD is rapidly distributed into highly vascularized organs including the liver and lungs and easily crosses the blood–brain barrier. Later, CBD is eliminated from vascularized tissue and sequestered in adipose tissue for up to several weeks (Lucas, Galettis and Schneider, 2018). There is a high volume of distribution of CBD reported at ~32 L/kg with sequestration into adipose tissue. Cytochrome P450 metabolism in the liver is mainly accomplished by CYP2C19 and CYP3A4 isoenzymes, resulting in the metabolite 7-hydroxy-CBD (Gaston *et al.*, 2017). Eventually the metabolites of CBD are eliminated largely in feces with some urinary metabolites.

Drug–Drug Interactions of CBD

Recent carefully conducted clinical trials of CBD in childhood epilepsy have reported significant drug–drug interactions (Geffrey *et al.*, 2015). In these trials that led to the approval of Epidiolex for Dravet syndrome (DS) and Lennox–Gastaut syndrome (LGS), CBD was found to elevate blood levels of the medication clobazam and its metabolite *N*-desmethylclobazam through the hepatic cytochrome P450 system. Clobazam is a benzodiazepine recently approved in the United States and was allowed to be prescribed in the Epidiolex clinical trials as a concomitant medication with CBD for DS and LGS epilepsy. Both CBD and clobazam are metabolized by 2C19 and coadministration of the medications inhibits the metabolism by CBD of clobazam and it's metabolite. CBD is also a potent inhibitor of additional cytochrome P450 isoenzymes including CYP2C9 and CYP3A4. Topiramate, metabolized by CYP2C9, and zonisamide, metabolized by CYP3A4, are additional anticonvulsants frequently used in the treatment of pediatric epilepsy. Both topiramate and zonisamide have been reported to demonstrate significant elevations in plasma when coadministered with CBD likely through the inhibition of the respective hepatic microenzyme systems.

Other anticonvulsants not metabolized by CYP2C19 and CYP2C9 have also been reported to be affected by coadministration with CBD. Rufinamide, a triazole derivative used to treat LGS, eslicarbazepine and oxcarbazepine have also been reported to be elevated in the presence of CBD (Gaston *et al.*, 2017). There is also a report of elevation in blood of the anticoagulant warfarin (Grayson *et al.*, 2018).

Finally, elevated liver enzymes have been reported in some patients treated with the coadministration of valproate and CBD. The authors noted in this report that the elevation of liver enzymes occurred without any change in valproate levels. Upon discontinuation of valproate and continuation with CBD the liver enzymes remained elevated (Gaston *et al.*, 2017).

Conversations to Have with Patients

In 2019 the World Health Organization (WHO) recommended to the United Nations (UN) that cannabis and its constituents be rescheduled to the least restrictive category. This would include marijuana, THC and CBD and essentially replace 60 years of restrictions applied to cannabis. Removing marijuana from the most restrictive schedule would reverse the position of the UN since 1961 and potentially encourage continuing relaxation of guidelines and possible legalization at the national level.

It can already be argued that this easing of restrictions and social acceptance is already well under way. In Canada and 47 states in the USA CBD containing less than 0.3% THC is already available. Sales of CBD in 2018 through health food stores in the USA was reported to exceed $52 billion and had a six-fold increase from the previous year. Slightly more restrictive guidelines exist in most parts of Europe with CBD available when derived from hemp with less than 0.2% THC. Sales of CBD in all distribution channels in Europe were estimated at $300 million with projections of 400% increase over the next several years. At the same time, other countries including Russia and China continue to limit possession and use of cannabis.

Despite the enormous expansion in the acceptance and use of CBD, limited scientific evidence supports the use and safety of this treatment in many conditions. Aside from the recent clinical trials of CBD in the treatment of two pediatric epilepsies and subsequent approval for use in the USA and EU, the clinician has limited information in advising patients. Misinformation and the growing belief that CBD is safe places further burdens on the clinicians that respond to their patients' questions about the drug.

Recently a study was published evaluating 84 samples of CBD oils, tinctures and liquids. Only 26 of the samples contained the reported amount of CBD and 18 were contaminated with THC. Many of the samples with CBD contained amounts lower than that reported in the label (Bonn-Miller *et al.*, 2017).

Other surveys on CBD are equally concerning. One report found that heavy metal contamination was present in the 10 leading brands of CBD sold with lead levels exceeding those reported in the unsafe drinking water of Flint, Michigan. Organophosphates known to be harmful to humans and amounts of CBD exceeding 700% of the labeled amount were found in these same leading brands of CBD further raising fears of public health hazards (Clean Label Project, 2019).

CBD is generally regarded as safe for use and this belief reassures patients that there are no concerns. The absence of psychoactive effects found with THC and the many benefits reported with CBD only reinforce the acceptance of the drug as a reasonable treatment. However, the lack of national standards and quality measurements for CBD clearly results in tainted products that may be unsafe to some individuals. Patients with preexisting illness including liver disease or concurrent medications are of special concern and should be monitored by their physician.

At the same time, CBD potentially offers enormous opportunity to better understand human afflictions and develop new treatments. Additional research into the effects of cannabinoids on non-cannabinoid receptors promises new discoveries and knowledge.

Bibliography

Adams, I. B. and Martin, B. R. (1996) 'Cannabis: pharmacology and toxicology in animals and humans', *Addiction*, 91(11), 1585–1614. doi:10.1046/j.1360-0443.1996.911115852.x.

Agurell, S. *et al.* (1986) 'Pharmacokinetics and metabolism of Δ1-tetrahydrocannabinol and other cannabinoids with emphasis on man', *Pharmacological Reviews*, 38(1), 21–43.

Bartner, L. R. *et al.* (2018) 'Pharmacokinetics of cannabidiol administered by 3 delivery methods at 2 different dosages to healthy dogs', *Canadian Journal of Veterinary Research*, 82(3), 178–183. Available at: www.ingentaconnect.com/content/cvma/cjvr/2018/00000082/00000003/art00002.

Bonn-Miller, M. O. *et al.* (2017). 'Labeling accuracy of cannabidiol extracts sold online', *JAMA: The Journal of the American Medical Association*, 318(17), 1708–1709. doi:10.1001/jama.2017.11909.

Brenneisen, R. (2007) 'Chemistry and analysis of phytocannabinoids and other cannabis constituents', in *Marijuana and the Cannabinoids*. Totowa: Humana Press, pp. 17–49. doi:10.1007/978-1-59259-947-9_2.

Brown, A. J. (2009) 'Novel cannabinoid receptors', *British Journal of Pharmacology*, 152(5), 567–575. doi:10.1038/sj.bjp.0707481.

Burstein, S., Rosenfeld, J. and Wittstruck, T. (1972) 'Isolation and characterization of two major urinary metabolites of Dgr1-tetrahydrocannabinol', *Science*, 176 (4033), 422–423. doi:10.1126/science.176.4033.422.

Clean Label Project (2019) https://cleanlabelproject.org/ (Accessed: December 1, 2019).

De Petrocellis, L. et al. (2012) 'Cannabinoid actions at TRPV channels: effects on TRPV3 and TRPV4 and their potential relevance to gastrointestinal inflammation', Acta Physiologica, 204(2), 255–266. doi:10.1111/j.1748-1716.2011.02338.x.

Gaoni, Y. and Mechoulam, R. (1964) 'Isolation, structure, and partial synthesis of an active constituent of hashish', Journal of the American Chemical Society, 86(8), 1646–1647. doi:10.1021/ja01062a046.

Gaston, T. E. et al. (2017) 'Interactions between cannabidiol and commonly used antiepileptic drugs', Epilepsia, 58(9), 1586–1592. doi:10.1111/epi.13852.

Geffrey, A. L. et al. (2015) 'Drug-drug interaction between clobazam and cannabidiol in children with refractory epilepsy', Epilepsia, 56(8), 1246–1251. doi:10.1111/epi.13060.

Gonca, E. and Darıcı, F. (2015) 'The effect of cannabidiol on ischemia/reperfusion-induced ventricular arrhythmias', Journal of Cardiovascular Pharmacology and Therapeutics, 20(1), 76–83. doi:10.1177/1074248414532013.

Grayson, L. et al. (2018) 'An interaction between warfarin and cannabidiol, a case report.', Epilepsy & Behavior Case Reports, 9, 10–11. doi:10.1016/j.ebcr.2017.10.001.

Greenberg, H. S. et al. (1994) 'Short-term effects of smoking marijuana on balance in patients with multiple sclerosis and normal volunteers', Clinical Pharmacology & Therapeutics, 55(3), 324–328. doi:10.1038/clpt.1994.33.

Gregg, L. C. et al. (2012). 'Activation of type 5 metabotropic glutamate receptors and diacylglycerol lipase-α initiates 2-arachidonoylglycerol formation and endocannabinoid-mediated analgesia', Journal of Neuroscience, 32(28), 9457–9468. doi:10.1523/JNEUROSCI.0013-12.2012.

Grotenhermen, F. (2002) 'The medical use of cannabis in Germany', Journal of Drug Issues, 32(2), 607–634. doi:10.1177/002204260203200218.

Grotenhermen, F. (2003) 'Pharmacokinetics and pharmacodynamics of cannabinoids', Clinical Pharmacokinetics, 42(4), 327–360. doi:10.2165/00003088-200342040-00003.

Halldin, M. M. et al. (1982) 'Urinary metabolites of delta 1-tetrahydrocannabinol in man.', Arzneimittel-Forschung, 32(7), 764–8. Available at: www.ncbi.nlm.nih.gov/pubmed/6289845.

Harvey, D. J. (1999) 'Absorption, distribution, and biotransformation of the cannabinoids', in Marihuana and Medicine. Totowa: Humana Press, pp. 91–103. doi:10.1007/978-1-59259-710-9_10.

Harvey, D. J. and Mechoulam, R. (1990) 'Metabolites of cannabidiol identified in human urine', Xenobiotica, 20(3), 303–320. doi:10.3109/00498259009046849.

Harvey, D. J., Samara, E. and Mechoulam, R. (1991) 'Comparative metabolism of cannabidiol in dog, rat and man', Pharmacology Biochemistry and Behavior, 40 (3), 523–532. doi:10.1016/0091-3057(91)90358-9.

Hawksworth, G. and McArdle, K. (2004) 'Metabolism and pharmacokinetics of cannabinoids', in G. Guy, B. Whittle and P. Robson (eds.), The Medicinal Uses of Cannabis and Cannabinoids. London: London Pharmaceutical Press. pp. 205–228.

Hejazi, N. et al. (2006) 'Δ9-Tetrahydrocannabinol and endogenous cannabinoid anandamide directly potentiate the function of glycine receptors', Molecular Pharmacology, 69(3), 991–997. doi:10.1124/mol.105.019174.

Hinz, B. and Ramer, R. (2019) 'Anti-tumour actions of cannabinoids', British Journal of Pharmacology, 176(10), 1384–1394. doi:10.1111/bph.14426.

Huestis, M. A. (2007) 'Human cannabinoid pharmacokinetics', Chemistry and Biodiversity, 4(8), 1770–1804. doi:10.1002/cbdv.200790152.

Ibeas Bih, C. et al. (2015) 'Molecular targets of cannabidiol in neurological disorders', Neurotherapeutics, 12(4), 699–730. doi:10.1007/s13311-015-0377-3.

Jiang, R. et al. (2011) 'Identification of cytochrome P450 enzymes responsible for metabolism of cannabidiol by human liver microsomes', *Life Sciences*, 89(5–6), 165–170. doi:10.1016/j.lfs.2011.05.018.

Kathmann, M. *et al.* (2006) 'Cannabidiol is an allosteric modulator at mu- and delta-opioid receptors', *Naunyn-Schmiedeberg's Archives of Pharmacology*, 372(5), 354–361. doi:10.1007/s00210-006-0033-x.

Lauckner, J. *et al.* (2008) 'GPR55 is a cannabinoid receptor that increases intracellular calcium and inhibits M current', *Proceedings of the National Academy of Sciences of the United States of America*, 105 (7), 2699–2704. Available at: www.pnas.org/content/105/7/2699.short.

Lucas, C. J., Galettis, P. and Schneider, J. (2018) 'The pharmacokinetics and the pharmacodynamics of cannabinoids', *British Journal of Clinical Pharmacology*, 84(11), 2477–2482. doi:10.1111/bcp.13710.

Mahgoub, M. *et al.* (2013) 'Effects of cannabidiol on the function of α7-nicotinic acetylcholine receptors', *European Journal of Pharmacology*, 720(1–3), 310–319. doi:10.1016/j.ejphar.2013.10.011.

Martin, B. R. *et al.* (1991) 'Behavioral, biochemical, and molecular modeling evaluations of cannabinoid analogs', *Pharmacology Biochemistry and Behavior*, 40 (3), 471–478. doi:10.1016/0091-3057(91) 90349-7.

McHugh, D. *et al.* (2012) 'Δ9-Tetrahydrocannabinol and N-arachidonyl glycine are full agonists at GPR18 receptors and induce migration in human endometrial HEC-1B cells', *British Journal of Pharmacology*, 165(8), 2414–2424. doi:10.1111/j.1476-5381.2011.01497.x.

Millar, S. A. *et al.* (2018) 'A systematic review on the pharmacokinetics of cannabidiol in humans', *Frontiers in Pharmacology*, 9, 1365. doi:10.3389/fphar.2018.01365.

Moreno-Navarrete, J. M. *et al.* (2012) 'The L-α-lysophosphatidylinositol/GPR55 system and its potential role in human obesity.', *Diabetes*, 61(2), 281–291. doi:10.2337/db11-0649.

Newmeyer, M. N. *et al.* (2016) 'Free and glucuronide whole blood cannabinoids' pharmacokinetics after controlled smoked, vaporized, and oral cannabis administration in frequent and occasional cannabis users: identification of recent cannabis intake', *Clinical Chemistry*, 62 (12), 1579–1592. doi:10.1373/clinchem.2016.263475.

Ohlsson, A. *et al.* (1986) 'Single-dose kinetics of deuterium-labelled cannabidiol in man after smoking and intravenous administration', *Biological Mass Spectrometry*, 13(2), 77–83. doi:10.1002/bms.1200130206.

O'Sullivan, S. E. (2007) 'Cannabinoids go nuclear: evidence for activation of peroxisome proliferator-activated receptors', *British Journal of Pharmacology*, 152(5), 576–582. doi:10.1038/sj.bjp.0707423.

Penumarti, A. and Abdel-Rahman, A. A. (2014) 'The novel endocannabinoid receptor GPR18 is expressed in the rostral ventrolateral medulla and exerts tonic restraining influence on blood pressure', *Journal of Pharmacology and Experimental Therapeutics*, 349(4), 29–38. doi:10.1124/jpet.113.209213.

Pertwee, RG. *et al.* (2010) 'International Union of Basic and Clinical Pharmacology. LXXIX. Cannabinoid receptors and their ligands: beyond CB₁ and CB₂', *Pharmacological Reviews*, 62(4), 588–631. doi:10.1124/pr.110.003004.588.

Pistis, M. and O'Sullivan, S. E. (2017) 'The role of nuclear hormone receptors in cannabinoid function', *Advances in Pharmacology*, 80, 291–328. doi:10.1016/bs.apha.2017.03.008.

Ramer, R. *et al.* (2013) 'COX-2 and PPAR-γ confer cannabidiol-induced apoptosis of human lung cancer cells', *Molecular Cancer Therapeutics*, 12(1), 69–82. doi:10.1158/1535-7163.MCT-12-0335.

Russo, E. B. *et al.* (2005). 'Agonistic properties of cannabidiol at 5-HT1a receptors', *Neurochemical Research*, 30(8), 1037–1043. doi:10.1007/s11064-005-6978-1.

Ryberg, E. *et al.* (2009) 'The orphan receptor GPR55 is a novel cannabinoid receptor', *British Journal of Pharmacology*, 152(7), 1092–1101. doi:10.1038/sj.bjp.0707460.

Sagredo, O. *et al.* (2007) 'Cannabinoids and neuroprotection in basal ganglia disorders', *Molecular Neurobiology*, 36(1), 82–91. doi:10.1007/s12035-007-0004-3.

Sagredo, O. *et al.* (2011) 'Neuroprotective effects of phytocannabinoid-based medicines in experimental models of Huntington's disease', *Journal of Neuroscience Research*, 89 (9), 1509–1518. doi:10.1002/jnr.22682.

Stinchcomb, A. L. *et al.* (2004) 'Human skin permeation of Δ^8-tetrahydrocannabinol, cannabidiol and cannabinol', *Journal of Pharmacy and Pharmacology*, 56(3), 291–297. doi:10.1211/0022357022791.

Stout, S. M. and Cimino, N. M. (2014) 'Exogenous cannabinoids as substrates, inhibitors, and inducers of human drug metabolizing enzymes: a systematic review', *Drug Metabolism Reviews*, 46(1), 86–95. doi:10.3109/03602532.2013.849268.

Xiong, W. *et al.* (2012) 'Cannabinoids suppress inflammatory and neuropathic pain by targeting α3 glycine receptors', *Journal of Experimental Medicine*, 209(6), 1121–1134. doi:10.1084/jem.20120242.

Yamaori, S. *et al.* (2010) 'Characterization of major phytocannabinoids, cannabidiol and cannabinol, as isoform-selective and potent inhibitors of human CYP1 enzymes', *Biochemical Pharmacology*, 79 (11), 1691–1698. doi:10.1016/j. bcp.2010.01.028.

The Endocannabinoids

The best and most efficient pharmacy is within your own system.
Robert Peale

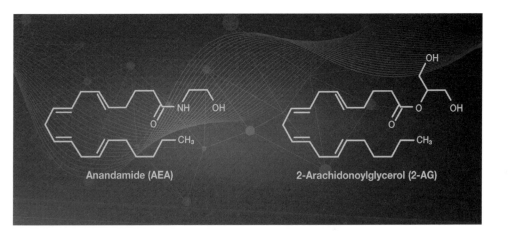

Anandamide (AEA) 2-Arachidonoylglycerol (2-AG)

- The endocannabinoid system consists of two cannabinoid receptors (cannabinoid receptor 1 [CB_1] and cannabinoid receptor 2 [CB_2]), two endocannabinoids (2-arachidonoylglycerol [2-AG] and N-arachidonoylethanolamine [anandamide; AEA]) and associated enzymatic processes for biosynthesis and degradation of endocannabinoids.
- CB_1 and CB_2 are in the G protein-coupled receptor (GPCR) family found in the central and peripheral systems. GPCRs including CB_1 and CB_2 function as binding sites for numerous drugs that act on the brain and peripheral nervous system.
- 2-AG is a *full agonist* at both CB_1 and CB_2 receptors. The concentration of 2-AG and distribution within the central nervous system is greater than AEA. 2-AG is the primary active endocannabinoid.
- AEA is a *partial agonist* at both CB_1 and CB_2 receptors and TRPV1.
- Endocannabinoids generally act through *retrograde* transmission to the CB_1 receptor on the presynaptic cell and inhibit neurotransmitter release.

- AEA and 2-AG are synthesized on demand in response and, unlike neurotransmitters, are not stored in vesicles.
- AEA biosynthesis may involve multiple pathways and degradation while 2-AG biosynthesis is generally through hydrolysis of 2-arachidonate diacylglycerols.
- Both AEA and 2-AG are rapidly removed from the synaptic cleft and degraded in a two-step process by fatty acid amide hydrolase (FAAH) and monoacylglycerol lipase (MAGL) respectively.

Introduction

As we have discussed previously in Chapters 1 and 2, cannabinoids have been very difficult to isolate and study due to their significant lipophilic properties. Once it was finally determined that $(-)\Delta^9$-tetrahydrocannabinol (THC) was the psychoactive component in cannabis (Gaoni and Mechoulam, 1964), attention quickly focused on understanding how THC worked in the brain. Many believed cannabinoids acted directly on membranes and did not bind specifically to receptors because of the high lipophilicity of THC.

Within a few years, the activity of THC was surprisingly found to be stereospecific with the psychoactive properties expressed only with the (-) isomer of the molecule. This implied that a specific cellular target accounted for the physiological effects of THC and other phytocannabinoids (Gaoni and Mechoulam, 1964). After more hydrophilic, synthetically modified radioligands of THC were available a closer analysis of the actions of cannabinoids on cell membranes could then be undertaken. Using these new techniques, a specific receptor was found in the rat brain that bound (-) isomer of THC (Devane et al., 1988). This receptor was named cannabinoid receptor 1 (CB_1) and was subsequently cloned two years later (Matsuda et al., 1990). Following this work, a second receptor was quickly discovered and also cloned from the canine intestine (Munro, Thomas and Abu-Shaar, 1993) and was named cannabinoid receptor 2 (CB_2). Over the past 25 years the search for other cannabinoid receptors has continued and several candidates have been proposed. However, only CB_1 and CB_2 are established as cannabinoid receptors.

The discovery of the CB_1 and CB_2 receptors raised the obvious question why the brain would contain specific targets for the plant-based cannabinoids. A similar issue had arisen a few years earlier with the discovery of the opiate receptor in the brain that bound plant-based opiate molecules from opium. Eventually the endorphin system was identified, which consisted of a family of opiate receptors and their endogenous agonists in addition to synthetic and degradative pathways (Mechoulam and Parker, 2013).

In a similar fashion, once the cannabinoid receptors had been isolated, research proceeded to answer why they were present in the body and how they function. Over the ensuing years naturally occurring ligands termed endocannabinoids were found and their biosynthetic and degradative pathways identified. Collectively, the cannabinoid receptors, the endocannabinoids and their associated enzymatic process are now referred to as the endocannabinoid system (ECS)(Mechoulam and Parker, 2013). Although much is now known about the constituent parts of the ECS, understanding the complex physiological mechanisms and their purpose remains a puzzle yet to be answered.

Both CB_1 and CB_2 are members of the G protein-coupled receptor (GPCR) superfamily. GPCRs are the largest known class of membrane receptors in eukaryotes with over 1000 separate types identified in humans. Many of the medications used in central nervous system (CNS) disorders act on GPCRs and these targets provide molecular targets for approximately half of medications currently in use (Höller, Freissmuth and Nanoff, 1999).

All GPCRs including CB_1 and CB_2 are transmembrane receptors coupled with guanine nucleotide binding proteins that bind neurotransmitters. Each receptor has an N-terminus tail extending into the extracellular space and a C-terminus within the cytoplasm. The receptor has a seven-transmembrane hydrophobic structure and typically couples with the G protein at the third membrane crossing. Each receptor usually binds to one or only a few molecules and serves a single function within the body. In the CNS, the GPCRs are the most numerous receptors present and serve a central role in the chemical signaling between cells.

Binding of neurotransmitters in the synaptic cleft to the N-terminus initiates intracellular activity and activates membrane-anchored adenyl cyclase with conversion of adenosine triphosphate (ATP) to cyclic adenosine monophosphate (cAMP). Through this process, the neurotransmitter in the synaptic cleft activates intracellularly the second messenger system of cAMP and triggers a cascade of intracellular events (Collins, Caron and Lefkowitz, 1992; Carman and Benovic, 1998).

GPCRs are heterotrimer proteins consisting of α, β and γ subunits with a great deal of complexity. The α subunits are much more heterogeneous when compared with the greater similarity between the other two subunits. When a ligand binds to the receptor, conformational changes occur that allow the α subunit to associate with the receptor and disassociate from the β and γ subunits. Through these changes intracellular changes are induced (Rodbell, 1997).

CB$_1$ and CB$_2$ are GPCRs that are strongly expressed in the basal ganglia and cerebellum with lesser concentration in the hippocampus layers I and IV within the cerebral cortex (Elphick and Egertova, 2001; Pertwee and Ross, 2002). When ligands bind to the cannabinoid receptors, conformational changes in the G protein inhibit adenyl cyclase and either inhibit voltage-gated Ca^{2+} channels or open K^+ inward channels. These structural and ion channel changes result in diverse and complex molecular processes within the cell through phosphorylation via second messenger systems and release of neurotransmitters contained within presynaptic vesicles is inhibited (Basavarajappa, 2017).

Activation of the CB$_1$ and CB$_2$ receptors initiates complex processes within the presynaptic cell. These result in inhibition of neurotransmitters that may be excitatory or inhibitory, and many of the resultant physiological effects are yet to be discovered. Behavior, immune function, growth factors, smell, taste and vision are among some of the many functions mediated by the GPCR superfamily and cannabinoids are the most widely expressed member with many potentially beneficial effects unknown at present.

The Cannabinoid Receptors CB$_1$ and CB$_2$

CB$_1$ was first found in the CNS and this led to the mistaken belief that the receptor was limited to the brain. CB$_2$, later discovered in the spleen, similarly was incorrectly thought to be a peripheral receptor only and limited to interaction with the immune system. Only after additional studies, however, was it accepted that CB$_1$ and CB$_2$ receptors are expressed in different concentrations in both central and peripheral locations (Howlett, 1998).

CB$_1$ is the receptor through which the phytocannabinoid THC asserts its psychoactive effects. It is by far the most prevalent cannabinoid receptor in the body with the highest density within the CNS. In the rodent brain, the CB$_1$ receptor is highly expressed in the basal ganglia and cerebellum and, to a lesser extent, over centers including the hippocampus and amygdala and some layers of the cerebral cortex. The CB$_1$ receptor is also found in multiple locations outside the CNS including heart, vascular, intestinal, immune cells and testes (Pertwee, 1999; Mackie, 2005, 2008) indicating the many functions the receptor serves.

There is a remarkable similarity in the CB$_1$ receptor across species with a similar amino acid sequence within mammals of 97–99%. There is also a significant homology in the amino acid sequences between the CB$_1$ and CB$_2$ receptors suggesting a shared genetic origin between the two cannabinoid receptors that has been conserved through evolution (Onaivi et al., 2002).

Although the CB_1 receptor inhibits neurotransmitter release and mediates intercellular communication, CB_1 receptors are found primarily on intracellular organelles including mitochondria, endoplasmic reticulum and tubules. When the cell is activated through propagation of the action potential and influx of Ca^{2+}, the number of membrane CB_1 receptors are greatly increased. There are examples of small ligands, such as nitrous oxide, that permeate cellular membranes and bind only to intracellular receptors but, in general, non-cannabinoid GPCRs are located typically on cell membranes. Only when these membrane GPCRs are activated during agonist activity is expression of the surface receptors increased. Phytocannabinoids, in part because of the high lipophilic properties, may also directly stimulate these intracellular cannabinoid receptors before full activation of the cell occurs.

The CB_1 receptor is remarkable in that it actually consists of two binding sites referred to as the orthosteric and allosteric sites. The orthosteric site serves as the main binding component for most cannabinoid agonists including THC while the adjacent allosteric site is secondary to other molecules (Neubig *et al.*, 2003). Molecules binding to the allosteric site exert conformational changes on the allosteric site and can significantly influence the binding properties of the main site (Christopoulos and Kanakin, 2002). The CB_2 receptor is believed by some to also possess orthosteric and allosteric binding sites although this is less well determined.

Changes in the binding properties of the orthosteric site through influence from the adjacent allosteric site are of considerable interest. Future therapeutic agents could be developed that potentially alter the binding of THC and the unwanted psychoactive properties. Allosteric agonists generally demonstrate activity only in the presence of molecules binding to the orthosteric site. In addition, there is usually greater variation in the structure of the orthosteric site proving multiple receptor subtypes available for pharmaceutical manipulation and development (Nguyen *et al.*, 2018).

Other phytocannabinoids may also bind to the allosteric site. Most important, the phytocannabinoid cannabidiol (CBD) is a weak agonist at the allosteric site but has no affinity for the orthosteric site that binds other cannabinoids. This indirect effect of CBD may eventually provide important mitigation of the psychoactive effects of THC and other molecules with significant adverse properties.

Information about the CB_2 receptor is much less conclusive than that about the CB_1 receptor. Although it was first identified in spleen and circulating lymphocytes, it is now established that it is present in both peripheral and central sites including in microglia, monocytes, mast cells, B-lymphocytes and microglia and astrocytes within the CNS (Onaivi *et al.*, 2012). Unlike CB_1, the CB_2 receptor has limited immunogenicity and is difficult to detect using classical antibody techniques. In addition, CB_1 receptors are highly expressed in the CNS and numerous peripheral sites while expression of CB_2 is less abundant but highly inducible (Maresz *et al.*, 2005). Similar to the CB_1 receptor, the CB_2 receptor is coupled to the $G_{i/o}$ protein and, when occupied by a ligand, inhibits adenyl cyclase and activates mitogen-activated protein (MAP) kinases. Potentially, manipulation of the CB_2 receptor may play important roles in multiple processes including inflammation, osteoporosis, cancer and neuropsychiatric conditions such as anxiety and addiction.

Some have speculated that the CB_2 receptor might be part of a protective system for the body against nonprotein invasion and injury (Pacher and Mechoulam, 2012). Supportive of this belief is the observation that the CB_2 receptor has affinity for endocannabinoids and other receptor agonists in response to many pathological conditions where injury to tissue is limited including cardiovascular, neurodegenerative, neuropsychiatric and pain.

The Endocannabinoids

The endocannabinoids are derived from arachidonic acid and are lipid messengers present in the CNS and peripheral nervous system. Only two known endocannabinoids, N-arachidonoylethanolamide (AEA or anandamide) and 2-arachidonoylglycerol (2-AG), have been identified and others may yet be discovered. Both lipid messengers are polyunsaturated fatty acids derived from arachidonic acid. Although endocannabinoids serve multiple roles in chemical messaging between neurons, they differ significantly from the classic neurotransmitters such as the monoamines and acetylcholine. One important difference is that endocannabinoids are highly hydrophobic, are produced only upon demand rather than stored in vesicles, only at the local, activated postsynaptic neuron, and traverse the synaptic cleft in a retrograde direction and bind to the CB_1 and CB_2 receptors on the presynaptic cell. After binding they are quickly removed, within a few milliseconds, from the synaptic cleft through an unidentified uptake mechanism, thus terminating the chemical communication. In comparison, phytocannabinoids including THC bind to all of their potential receptors and can remain active for an extended time. Thus, plant-based cannabinoids have a broad, enduring effect on intercellular communication. Endocannabinoids have a more limited and targeted effect similar to other neurotransmitters that are rapidly terminated.

This retrograde transmission by lipid messengers is a key concept to understand how cannabinoids modulate intercellular communication. Endocannabinoids inhibit the release of both excitatory and inhibitory neurotransmitters and, dependent upon the neurotransmitter, inhibit or stimulate the postsynaptic cell. For example, glutamate, the most prominent excitatory neurotransmitter in the brain, and gamma-aminobutyric acid (GABA), the most frequent inhibitory neurotransmitter, are both modulated by the endocannabinoids. Dopamine, serotonin and norepinephrine, although less abundant, bind to GPCRs and interact with cannabinoids.

AEA was the first endocannabinoid discovered in 1992 and is found in the CNS and peripheral tissue (Devane et al., 1992; Zoerner et al., 2011). Initially, AEA was isolated from porcine brain and found to be present in the CNS at amounts similar to the neurotransmitters dopamine and serotonin.

The CB_1 receptor is the most prominent cannabinoid receptor in the body but the distribution of AEA is not closely associated with that of the receptor. When binding to the receptor, AEA is also only a partial agonist at the binding site. This disparity in the localization of the CB_1 receptor and AEA plus limited binding affinity suggest additional roles for this endocannabinoid (Pertwee et al., 2010).

2-AG was the second endocannabinoid discovered and was also isolated in brain tissue (Mechoulam et al., 1995). Exactly as with AEA, 2-AG is a derivative of arachidonic acid and is synthesized on demand upon the activation of the cell through increase of intracellular calcium. Unlike AEA, 2-AG is present in considerably larger amounts in the CNS and is a full agonist at both the CB_1 receptor and the CB_2 receptor (Sugiura et al., 2002; Pertwee et al., 2010).

Both AEA and 2-AG are classified as endocannabinoids, but other molecules are sometimes referred to as "like endocannabinoids" as well. Omega-6 derivatives, noladin ether (2-arachidonoyl glyceryl ether) (Hanus et al., 2001), virodhamine (Porter et al., 2002) and N-arachidonoyl dopamine (NADA) (Huang et al., 2002) also bind to the CB_1 and CB_2 receptors with different affinities although they are not identified as classic endocannabinoids.

Non-cannabinoid Receptors Influenced by Cannabinoids

Receptors other than CB_1 and CB_2 also bind phytocannabinoids and endocannabinoids. Although affinity for the CB_1 and CB_2 is a property shared by AEA and 2-AG, both endocannabinoids also bind to multiple targets other than cannabinoid receptors. Lipid signaling systems are well known to bind multiple ligands and the endocannabinoids are not limited only to CB_1 and CB_2 receptors.

Transient Receptor Potential Channels

Transient receptor potential (TRP) channels are a family of nonselective cation channel receptors that influence the membrane permeability of sodium, calcium and magnesium. A remarkable range of stimuli influence the TRP family of receptors and include temperature, touch and pressure, light, taste and olfaction.

TRPV1 was the first TRP channel to be identified and is a postsynaptic receptor located on the cytosol-facing inner membrane of the cell. TRPV1 is present not only in sensory neurons but also other tissue including epithelial, endothelial, muscle and lymphocytes (Starowicz, Nigam and Di Marzo, 2007). This receptor also is found to dimerize with CB_1 receptors in dorsal root and spinal cord tissue resulting in complex cellular communication (Ahluwalia *et al.*, 2003). Capsaicin (chili pepper), allicin (garlic) and allyl isothiocyanate (wasabi and horseradish) are among the many stimuli known to activate TRPV. Heat and pain also activate the TRPV1 channel and this receptor is sometimes referred to as vanilloid and is an important modulator in the perception of pain and nociception. AEA and the phytocannabinoids THC and CBD are full agonists at the TRPV1 receptor.

Since the TRPV1 receptor is located within the inner layer of the postsynaptic cell, AEA binds intracellularly to this receptor. In contrast AEA binds to cannabinoid receptors after retrograde transmission across the synapse (Alger, 2002). Other molecules including the non-cannabinoid NADA (Huang *et al.*, 2002) are also full agonists in addition to other phytocannabinoids including CBD and THC (De Petrocellis *et al.*, 2011; Morales, Reggio and Jagerovic, 2017). In contrast, 2-AG, a full agonist for CB_1 and CB_2 receptors, apparently has no affinity for the TRPV1 site.

At least five additional TRPV channels have been identified. None of these TRPV receptors bind capsaicin but collectively this remaining family of receptors respond to a variety of temperature, pain and pressure stimuli (Pertwee *et al.*, 2010).

G Protein Receptor 55

GPR55 was discovered in 1999 (Sawzdargo *et al.*, 1999) and initially believed to be a third cannabinoid receptor (Moriconi *et al.*, 2010) although later work demonstrated little sequence similarity between this receptor and CB_1 and CB_2 (McPartland *et al.*, 2006b). However, all three are GPCRs and GPR55 is highly expressed in the large dorsal root ganglion. Activation of GPR55 increases with inflow of Ca^{2+} and AEA is a partial agonist at this receptor. Other pharmacological activity at GPR55 is complex with little agreement to date. Compounds known to activate CB_1 and or CB_2 (such as 2-AG and THC) apparently have inconsistent findings or no effect on this receptor (Lauckner *et al.*, 2008).

AEA, in contrast, in some studies has been reported to have a greater potency for GPR55 when compared with its affinity for CB_1 and CB_2 (Lauckner *et al.*, 2008; Henstridge *et al.*,

2009). In other studies, AEA has been inconsistent with differences dependent upon dosage and assay. Although the role of AEA as a ligand for GPR55 remains controversial, there is greater agreement that 2-AG has little interaction with this receptor.

Of great interest is the finding that GPR55 is blocked by the phytocannabinoid CBD. The receptor is located on excitatory glutamate neurons and the antagonistic actions of CBD on this receptor may play a critical role in seizure and eating disorders (*Sylantyev et al.*, 2013; Parker, 2017).

Peroxisome Proliferator-Activated Receptor (PPAR)

PPAR proteins are three isoforms (PPARα, PPARγ and PPARβ/δ) within a family of nuclear hormone receptors activated by lipid molecules. These receptors are not activated by any single ligand but are instead regarded as lipid sensors and that respond to changes in metabolism. As endocannabinoids are derivatives of a fatty acid, both AEA and 2-AG are agonists of at least two PPAR isoforms. Once activated, the proteins become transcription factors that regulate metabolism and cellular differentiation through regulation of gene expression in the nucleus (Michalik *et al.*, 2006). PPARs are found in skeletal muscle, endothelium, adipose tissue and liver to differing degrees (Pertwee *et al.*, 2010). When activated, PPARs regulate gene expression, inflammatory response especially in the cardiovascular system, cell growth and differentiation and apoptosis. When activated, PPAR also decreases the inflammatory response in the cardiovascular system and endothelium (Duan, Usher and Mortensen, 2009; Cantini *et al.*, 2010).

The Biosynthesis and Degradation of Endocannabinoids

As previously discussed, endocannabinoids are highly lipophilic and not stored in vesicles. Unlike the typical neurotransmitter that is stored in vesicles, endocannabinoids are produced within the activated cell "on demand" by depolarization of the postsynaptic neuron and the influx of Ca^{2+}. Although both AEA and 2-AG are synthesized from arachidonic acid embedded in the postsynaptic membrane, each endocannabinoid undergoes separate pathways for biosynthesis and biodegradation.

The biosynthesis of AEA is a two-step process that can proceed through multiple pathways. Phosphatidylethanolamine (PE) is a major phospholipid constituent of biological membranes that serves as the precursor for the synthesis of AEA. Through the action of the enzyme *N*-acetyltransferase, this phospholipid is converted into *N*-arachidonoyl-PE. The enzyme phospholipase D completes the process with the synthesis of AEA and phosphatidic acid (Piomelli, 2003).

Similar to AEA, 2-AG is produced "on demand" upon activation of the postsynaptic neuron.

Phosphatidylinositol, a membrane phospholipid, and arachidonic acid undergo enzymatic modification to produce 2-AG. 1,2-Diacylglycerol (DAG) is the immediate precursor to 2-AG. As with AEA, there are multiple pathways available for the synthesis and conversion of DAG to 2-AG. Hydrolysis by DAG lipase is currently considered the primary step in the biosynthesis of 2-AG (Sugiura *et al.*, 2002).

Endocannabinoids, like many neurotransmitters but unlike the exogenous phytocannabinoids, are quickly degraded, terminating the chemical messaging between cells. Hydrolysis is the major pathway of degradation although each endocannabinoid relies on different enzymatic pathways. AEA is degraded to arachidonic acid and ethanolamine by two postsynaptic, membrane-attached enzymes, fatty acid amide hydrolase (FAAH) 1 and 2 (Cravatt *et al.*, 1996). FAAH 1 and 2 are located in areas of high expression of the CB_1 receptor and found in higher concentrations in postsynaptic neurons. Once AEA is released from the presynaptic receptor, the molecule likely diffuses back across the synaptic cleft and is conveyed by an unidentified transport system into the post-synaptic cell, similar to other chemical messaging systems such as serotonergic and noradrenergic systems. Once inside the postsynaptic neuron, AEA is transported by proteins to FAAH attached to cytosol facing membrane locations and broken down to arachidonic acid and ethanolamine. Other less important pathways in addition to hydrolysis with FAAH are also available in the degradation of AEA. Instead of hydrolysis, AEA may also undergo oxidation by several families of enzymes including cyclooxy-genases (COX-1 and COX-2), lipoxygenases and epoxygenases. From this complicated oxidative process breaking down AEA, prostaglandin derivatives are formed (Hermanson *et al.*, 2013).

2-AG undergoes a similar breakdown process and can also be degraded through either hydrolysis or oxidative pathways. The primary route of degradation occurs in the presynaptic neuron with the enzyme monoacylglycerol lipase (Dinh, Kathuria, and Piomelli, 2004). FAAH may also break down 2-AG as a secondary hydrolysis in either presynaptic or postsynaptic neurons. Oxidation is also available but is a less important pathway of degradation utilizing COX-2 and lipoxygenase enzymes (Yates and Baker, 2009).

Retrograde Signaling by Endocannabinoids

Retrograde release of endocannabinoids on activation of the postsynaptic nerve is a unique property of the ECS. Other molecules are also known to influence the activity of the presynaptic cell including nitric acid and growth factors. (Davis and Murphey, 1994; Williams, 1996; Davis and Goodman, 1998; Regehr, Carey and Best, 2009). Retrograde signaling exhibits several properties that are especially characteristic of the ECS. First, synthesis and release from the postsynaptic neuron occurs after activation of the cell. Then follows a release of the endocannabinoid into the synaptic cleft potentially with the assistance of a yet to be identified transport system and binding to the presynaptic canna-binoid receptor. Finally, the release of neurotransmitter in the presynaptic cell is reduced and the consequences of the anterograde propagation of the signal altered (Figure 3.1) (Regehr, Carey and Best, 2009).

Retrograde Endocannabinoid Transmission

In 1994 this unique process of cellular communication was proposed by Devane and Axelrod (Devane, 1994; Devane and Axelrod, 1994). Subsequent work demonstrated that both excitatory and inhibitory properties of the presynaptic neurotransmitter could be inhibited. Thus, a short-term excitation would result by inhibition of GABA-containing neurons in a process termed depolarization-induced suppression of inhibition (DSI) (Llano, Leresche and Marty, 1991; Pitler and Alger, 1992). Later work also described depolarization-induced suppression of excitation (DSE) in glutamate-producing axons (Kreitzer and Regehr, 2001). DSI was shown to decrease the input of inhibitory cells for several seconds resulting in a fast retrograde effect. DSE was then later reported to have lasted several minutes following inhibition of the excitatory axon.

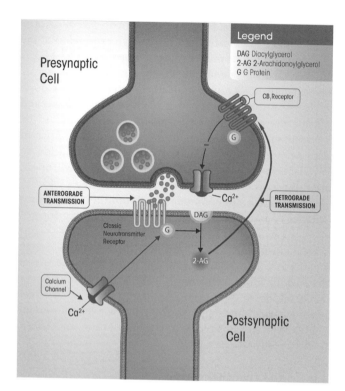

Figure 3.1 Retrograde signaling of endocannabinoids.

Concluding Thoughts

The identification of the CB_1 and CB_2 receptors and the discovery of the ECS are recent events that have all occurred since the 1980s. This research was driven by the curiosity to understand how *Cannabis sativa*, a plant used for thousands of years for religious, therapeutic and recreational purposes, worked in man.

In the quest to learn more about an ancient plant, medical science has accidentally uncovered a treasure containing unimagined secrets about life and health. The similarities between the effects of cannabis and the endocannabinoids are unfortunately used by some to demonstrate equivalency between the two. But this belief could not be further from the truth.

The genus *Cannabis* likely originated long before human history in central Asia. Over the millennia, the plant thrived and evolved into different species suited for the diverse climates of earth. Phytocannabinoids, constituents of *C. sativa*, also were conserved perhaps as part of evolutionary adaption for survival.

It would not be surprising if *C. sativa* evolved phytocannabinoids to protect the plant from predators. In the past, cannabis has been used as a pesticide and fungicide for centuries perhaps demonstrating the toxicity to potential threats.

Endocannabinoids evolved throughout the animal kingdom in close association with the development of the cannabinoid receptors (McPartland *et al.*, 2006a, 2006b). Both AEA and 2-AG and CB_1 and CB_2 receptors have been found in vertebrate species and endocannabinoids have been reported in some invertebrate species as well.

Thus, phytocannabinoids evolved from the plant kingdom perhaps for a defensive role against attack. Within the animal kingdom another separate system named the ECS arose probably to enhance survival as well as unique to the needs of the organism. The molecules of plant and animal systems were dissimilar with significant differences in chemical signaling structure (three-ringed phytocannabinoids vs. long-chain fatty acids), affinity to cannabinoid receptors (THC and other phytocannabinoids are partial agonists while 2-AG is a full agonist), binding to non-cannabinoid receptors, half-life (prolonged in hours and days for phytocannabinoids vs. rapid in seconds and milliseconds for endocannabinoids) and site of action (activation of all receptors with affinity for the phytocannabinoids vs. discrete activation at limited location by endocannabinoids).

In later chapters we will discuss other differences in safety, tolerance and dependency of the phytocannabinoids and how they differ from endocannabinoids. As progress continues in understanding the actions of the ECS, undoubtedly greater knowledge of the body and potential novel treatments against disease may occur.

Bibliography

Ahluwalia, J. et al. (2003) 'Anandamide regulates neuropeptide release from capsaicin-sensitive primary sensory neurons by activating both the cannabinoid 1 receptor and the vanilloid receptor 1 in vitro', European Journal of Neuroscience, 17(12), 2611–2618. https://doi.org/10.1046/j.1460-9568.2003.02703.x.

Alger, B. E. (2002). 'Retrograde signalling in the regulation of synaptic transmission: focus on endocannabinoids', Progress in Neurobiology, 68(4), 247–286.

Basavarajappa, B. S. (2017) 'Cannabinoid receptors and their signaling mechanisms', in E. Murillo-Rodríguez (ed.), The Endocannabinoid System: Genetics, Biochemistry, Brain Disorders, and Therapy. London: Academic Press. pp. 25–62.

Cantini, G. et al. (2010) 'Peroxisome-proliferator-activated receptor gamma (PPARγ) is required for modulating endothelial inflammatory response through a nongenomic mechanism', European Journal of Cell Biology, 89(9), 645–653. https://doi.org/10.1016/j.ejcb.2010.04.002.

Carman, C. V and Benovic, J. L. (1998) 'G-protein-coupled receptors: turn-ons and turn-offs', Current Opinion in Neurobiology, 8(3), 335–344.

Christopoulos, A. and Kanakin, T. (2002). 'G protein-coupled receptor allosterism and complexing', Pharmacological Reviews, 54(2), 323–374.

Collins, S., Caron, M. G. and Lefkowitz, R. J. (1992) 'From ligand binding to gene expression: new insights into the regulation of G-protein-coupled receptors', Trends in Biochemical Sciences, 17(1), 37–39. https://doi.org/10.1016/0968-0004(92)90425-9.

Cravatt, B. F. et al. (1996) 'Molecular characterization of an enzyme that degrades neuromodulatory fatty-acid amides', Nature, 384(6604), 83–87. https://doi.org/10.1038/384083a0.

Davis, G. W. and Goodman, C. S. (1998) 'Synapse-specific control of synaptic efficacy at the terminals of a single neuron', Nature, 392(6671), 82–86. doi:10.1038/32176.

Davis, G. W. and Murphey, R. K. (1994) 'Retrograde signaling and the development of transmitter release properties in the invertebrate nervous system', Journal of Neurobiology, 25(6), 740–756. https://doi.org/10.1002/neu.480250612.

De Petrocellis, L. et al. (2011). 'Effects of cannabinoids and cannabinoid-enriched Cannabis extracts on TRP channels and endocannabinoid metabolic enzymes', British Journal of Pharmacology, 163, 1479–1494.

Devane, W. A. (1994) 'New dawn of cannabinoid pharmacology', Trends in Pharmacological Sciences, 15(2), 40–41. https://doi.org/10.1016/0165-6147(94)90106-6.

Devane, W. A. et al. (1988) 'Determination and characterization of a cannabinoid receptor in rat brain', *Molecular Pharmacology*, 34(5), 605–613.

Devane, W. A. *et al.* (1992) 'Isolation and structure of a brain constituent that binds to the cannabinoid receptor', *Science*, 258 (5090), 1946–1949. https://doi.org/10.1126/science.1470919.

Devane, W. A. and Axelrod, J. (1994) 'Enzymatic synthesis of anandamide, an endogenous ligand for the cannabinoid receptor, by brain membranes', *Proceedings of the National Academy of Sciences of the United States of America*, 91(14), 6698–6701. https://doi.org/10.1073/pnas.91.14.6698.

Dinh, T. P., Kathuria, S. and Piomelli, D. (2004) 'RNA interference suggests a primary role for monoacylglycerol lipase in the degradation of the endocannabinoid 2-arachidonoylglycerol', *Molecular Pharmacology*, 66(5), 1260–1264.

Duan, S. Z., Usher, M. G. and Mortensen, R. M. (2009) 'PPARs: the vasculature, inflammation and hypertension', *Current Opinion in Nephrology and Hypertension*, 18 (2), 128–133. https://doi.org/10.1097/MNH .0b013e328325803b.

Elphick, M. R. and Egertova, M. (2001) 'The neurobiology and evolution of cannabinoid signalling', *Philosophical Transactions of the Royal Society of London. Series B: Biological Sciences*, 356(1407), 381–408. https://doi.org /10.1098/rstb.2000.0787.

Gaoni, Y. and Mechoulam, R. (1964) 'Isolation, structure, and partial synthesis of an active constituent of hashish', *Journal of the American Chemical Society*, 86(8), 1646–1647. https://doi.org/10.1021 /ja01062a046.

Hanus, L. *et al.* (2001) '2-arachidonyl glyceryl ether, an endogenous agonist of the cannabinoid CB1 receptor', *Proceedings of the National Academy of Sciences of the United States of America*, 98, 3662–3665.

Henstridge, C. M., *et al.* (2009) 'The GPR55 ligand L-α-lysophosphatidylinositol promotes RhoA-dependent Ca^{2+} signaling and NFAT activation', *FASEB Journal*, 23(1), 183–193. https://doi.org/10.1096/fj.08 -108670.

Hermanson, D. J. *et al.* (2013) 'Substrate-selective COX-2 inhibition decreases anxiety via endocannabinoid activation', *Nature Neuroscience*, 16(9), 1291–1298. doi:10.1038/nn.3480.

Höller, C., Freissmuth, M. and Nanoff, C. (1999) 'G proteins as drug targets', *Cellular and Molecular Life Sciences CMLS*, 55(2), 257–270. https://doi.org/10.1007 /s000180050288.

Howlett, A. C. (1998) 'The CB_1 cannabinoid receptor in the brain', *Neurobiology of Disease*, 5(6), 405–416. https://doi.org/10 .1006/nbdi.1998.0215.

Huang, S. M. *et al.* (2002) 'An endogenous capsaicin-like substance with high potency at recombinant and native vanilloid VR1 receptors', *Proceedings of the National Academy of Sciences of the United States of America*, 99, 8400–8405.

Kreitzer, A. C. and Regehr, W. G. (2001) 'Retrograde inhibition of presynaptic calcium influx by endogenous cannabinoids at excitatory synapses onto Purkinje cells', *Neuron*, 29, 717–727. https://doi.org/10.1016 /S0896-6273(01)00246-X.

Lauckner, J. E. *et al.* (2008) 'GPR55 is a cannabinoid receptor that increases intracellular calcium and inhibits M current', *Proceedings of the National Academy of Sciences of the United States of America*, 105 (7), 2699–2704. https://doi.org/10.1073/pnas .0711278105.

Llano, I., Leresche, N. and Marty, A. (1991) 'Calcium entry increases the sensitivity of cerebellar purkinje cells to applied GABA and decreases inhibitory synaptic currents', *Neuron*, 6(4), 565–574. doi:10.1016/0896-6273(91)90059-9.

Mackie, K. (2005) 'Distribution of cannabinoid receptors in the central and peripheral nervous system', *Handbook of Experimental Pharmacology*, 168(1), 299–325. https://doi .org/10.1007/3-540-26573-2_10.

Mackie, K. (2008) 'Cannabinoid receptors: where they are and what they do', *Journal of Neuroendocrinology*, 20(s1), 10–14. https:// doi.org/10.1111/j.1365-2826.2008.01671.x.

Maresz, K. *et al.* (2005) 'Modulation of the cannabinoid CB_2 receptor in microglial cells in response to inflammatory stimuli', *Journal of Neurochemistry*, 95(2), 437–445. https://doi.org/10.1111/j.1471-4159.2005.03380.x.

Matsuda, L. A. *et al.* (1990). 'Structure of a cannabinoid receptor and functional expression of the cloned cDNA', *Nature*, 346, 561–564.

McPartland, J. M. et al. (2006a) 'Cannabinoid receptors in invertebrates', *Journal of Evolutionary Biology*, 19(2), 366–373. https://doi.org/10.1111/j.1420-9101.2005.01028.x.

McPartland, J. M. et al. (2006b) 'Evolutionary origins of the endocannabinoid system', *Gene*, 370(1–2), 64–74. https://doi.org/10.1016/j.gene.2005.11.004.

Mechoulam, R. *et al.* (1995) 'Identification of an endogenous 2-monoglyceride, present in canine gut, that binds to cannabinoid receptors', *Biochemical Pharmacology*, 50(1), 83–90. https://doi.org/10.1016/0006-2952(95)00109-D.

Mechoulam, R. and Parker, L. A. (2013) 'The endocannabinoid system and the brain', *Annual Review of Psychology*, 64, 21–47. https://doi.org/10.1146/annurev-psych-113011-143739.

Michalik, L. *et al.* (2006) 'International Union of Pharmacology. LXI. Peroxisome proliferator-activated receptors', *Pharmacological Reviews*, 58(4), 726–741. doi:10.1124/pr.58.4.5.

Morales, P., Reggio, P. H. and Jagerovic, N. (2017) 'An overview on medicinal chemistry of synthetic and natural derivatives of cannabidiol'. *Frontiers in Pharmacology*, 8, 422. https://doi.org/10.3389/fphar.2017.00422.

Moriconi, A. *et al.* (2010) 'GPR55: current knowledge and future perspectives of a purported cannabinoid receptor', *Current Medicinal Chemistry*, 17(14), 1411–1429. https://doi.org/10.2174/092986710790980069.

Munro, S., Thomas, K. L. and Abu-Shaar, M. (1993) 'Molecular characterization of the peripheral receptor for cannabinoids', *Nature*, 365(6441), 61–65.

Neubig, R. R. *et al.* (2003) 'International Union of Pharmacology Committee on Receptor Nomenclature and Drug Classification.

XXXVIII. Update on Terms and Symbols in Quantitative Pharmacology', *Pharmacological Reviews*, 55, 597–606.

Nguyen, T. *et al.* (2018) 'Allosteric modulation: an alternative approach targeting the cannabinoid CB1 receptor', *Medical Research Reviews*, 37(3), 441–474. https://doi.org/10.1002/med.21418.

Onaivi, E. S. *et al.* (2002) 'Endocannabinoids and cannabinoid receptor genetics', *Progress in Neurobiology*, 66(5), 307–344. https://doi.org/10.1016/S0301-0082(02)00007-2.

Onaivi, E. S. *et al.* (2012) 'CNS effects of CB2 cannabinoid receptors: beyond neuro-immuno-cannabinoid activity', *Journal of Psychopharmacology*, 26(1), 92–103.

Pacher, P. and Mechoulam, R. (2011) 'Is lipid signaling through cannabinoid 2 receptors part of a protective system?', *Progress in Lipid Research*, 50, 193–211.

Parker, L. A. (2017) *Cannabinoids and the Brain.* Cambridge, MA: MIT Press.

Pertwee, R. G. (1999) 'Evidence for the presence of CB_1 cannabinoid receptors on peripheral neurones and for the existence of neuronal non-CB_1 cannabinoid receptors', *Life Sciences*, 65(6–7), 597–605. https://doi.org/10.1016/S0024-3205(99)00282-9.

Pertwee, R. G. *et al.* (2010) 'International Union of Basic and Clinical Pharmacology. LXXIX. Cannabinoid receptors and their ligands: beyond CB_1 and CB_2', *Pharmacological Reviews*, 62(4), 588–631. https://doi.org/10.1124/pr.110.003004

Pertwee, R.G. and Ross, R. A. (2002) 'Cannabinoid receptors and their ligands', *Prostaglandins, Leukotrienes and Essential Fatty Acids*, 66(2–3), 101–121. https://doi.org/10.1054/plef.2001.0341

Piomelli, D. (2003) 'The molecular logic of endocannabinoid signalling', *Nature Reviews Neuroscience*, 4(11), 873–884. https://doi.org/10.1038/nrn1247.

Pitler, T. A. and Alger, B. E. (1992) 'Postsynaptic spike firing reduces synaptic GABAA responses in hippocampal pyramidal cells', *Journal of Neuroscience*, 12, 4122–4132. doi:10.1523/JNEUROSCI.12-10-04122.1992.

Porter, A. C. *et al.* (2002) 'Characterization of a novel endocannabinoid, virodhamine, with antagonist activity at the CB1 receptor', *Journal of Pharmacology and Experimental Therapeutics*, 301, 1020–1024.

Regehr, W. G., Carey, M. R. and Best, A. R. (2009) 'Activity-dependent regulation of synapses by retrograde messengers', *Neuron*, 63(2), 154–170. https://doi.org/10.1016/j.neuron.2009.06.021.

Rodbell, M. (1997) 'The complex regulation of receptor-coupled G-proteins', *Advances in Enzyme Regulation*, 37, 427–435. https://doi.org/10.1016/S0065-2571(96)00020-9.

Sawzdargo, M. *et al.* (1999) 'Identification and cloning of three novel human G protein-coupled receptor genes GPR52, PsiGPR53 and GPR55: GPR55 is extensively expressed in human brain', *Brain Research. Molecular Brain Research*, 64(2), 193–198. doi:10.1016/s0169-328x(98)00277-0.

Starowicz, K., Nigam, S. and Di Marzo, V. (2007) 'Biochemistry and pharmacology of endovanilloids', *Pharmacology & Therapeutics*, 114(1), 13–33. https://doi.org/10.1016/j.pharmthera.2007.01.005.

Sugiura, T. *et al.* (2002) 'Biosynthesis and degradation of anandamide and 2-arachidonoylglycerol and their possible significance', *Prostaglandins, Leukotrienes and Essential Fatty Acids*, 66, 173–192.

Sylantyev, S. *et al.* (2013) 'Cannabinoid- and lysophosphatidylinositol-sensitive receptor GPR55 boosts neurotransmitter release at central synapses', *Proceedings of the National Academy of Sciences of the United States of America*, 110(13), 5193–5198. doi:10.1073/pnas.1211204110.

Williams, J. H. (1996) 'Retrograde messengers and long-term potentiation: a progress report', *Journal of Lipid Mediators and Cell Signalling*, 14(1–3), 331–339.

Yates, M. L. and Barker, E. L. (2009) 'Inactivation and biotransformation of the endogenous cannabinoids anandamide and 2-arachidonoylglycerol', *Molecular Pharmacology*, 76(1), 11–17.

Zoerner, A. A. *et al.* (2011) 'Quantification of endocannabinoids in biological systems by chromatography and mass spectrometry: a comprehensive review from an analytical and biological perspective', *Biochimica et Biophysica Acta (BBA) – Molecular and Cell Biology of Lipids*, 1811(11), 706-723.

Approved Cannabinoid Medicines for Therapeutic Use

Medicine sometimes snatches away health, sometimes gives it.

Ovid, Tristia 2, 269

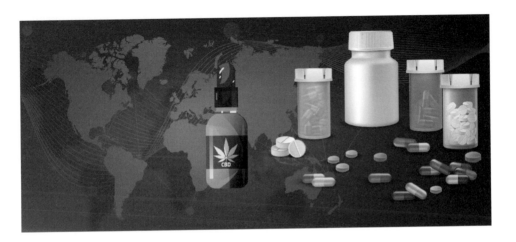

- Epidiolex (cannabidiol) is an extraction of cannabidiol (CBD) from *Cannabis sativa* first approved in 2018 in the USA and in the EU in 2019 for Lennox–Gastaut syndrome (LGS) and Dravet syndrome (DS) in children two years of age and older.
- Nabilone (Cesamet) is a synthetic analog of Δ^9-tetrahydrocannabinol (THC) first approved in the UK in 1985 for chemotherapy-induced nausea and vomiting (CINV).
- Dronabinol (Marinol and Syndros) is a synthetic THC first approved in the USA in 1985 for CINV and subsequently for anorexia associated with HIV in 1994. It is available in a soft gel capsule (Marinol) and liquid formulation (Syndros).
- Nabiximols (Sativex) is a combination of approximately 1:1 plant extraction of THC and CBD from *C. sativa* initially approved in the UK and Canada for pain related to spasticity.
- Access to medical marijuana is rapidly increasing in the USA, Canada, the UK and EU and other regions. Medical marijuana has not been scientifically reviewed by any regulatory agency and is not approved for any therapeutic use.

Introduction

The nineteenth and twentieth centuries witnessed advances in the ability to separate many biologically active molecules from plants and gave birth to the modern pharmaceutical industry. Even with today's current scientific advances with biotechnology and genomics, in the twenty-first century botanical extracts from plants continue to provide significant numbers of effective medicines. Cannabis, used for thousands of years, lagged behind this development, as described in Chapter 1, and only in 1985 were the first cannabinoid-based medicines approved. With the identification in the 1960s of $(-)\Delta^9$-tetrahydrocannabinol (THC) as the psychoactive component of *Cannabis sativa*, research into the properties of phytocannabinoids as potential new medicines actively began.

Since the first approvals in 1985, regulatory authorities in over 30 countries have now approved various products containing cannabinoids for prescription use. Five medicines are currently approved for prescription use but no one country has approved all five products (see Table 4.1). Both the USA (dronabinol [Syndros and Marinol], nabilone [Cesamet] and Epidiolex [cannabidiol]) and the European Union (EU) (dronabinol [Marinol], nabilone, nabiximols [Sativex] and Epidiolex) have approved four products with Canada (dronabinol [Marinol], nabilone and nabiximols) not too far behind. Some of the approved therapeutic indications for cannabinoid-based medications include chemotherapy-induced nausea and vomiting (CINV), anorexia associated with HIV, pain related to spasticity and two rare epilepsies in childhood.

To be approved, these medications were required to demonstrate efficacy and safety for the indication in adequately controlled, high-quality, randomized clinical trials (RCTs). Consistent standards of purity of the medication were required using the same standards applied to all approved medications. After approval, these cannabinoid-based medicines, like all prescription products, are continually monitored to ensure continuing safety and quality.

The first cannabinoid-based medicine to be approved was dronabinol in 1985 by the US Food and Drug Administration (FDA). Dronabinol is chemically synthesized THC in the laboratory and produced without any plant-derived constituents. It was originally approved for CINV and, several years later, for anorexia associated with HIV. It was initially available as a soft gel capsule under the brand name Marinol and subsequently in a liquid solution under the brand name Syndros. Nabilone, the second approved cannabinoid-based product, is an oral synthetic analog of THC also devoid of any plant constituents and originally approved for CINV. Nabiximols, marketed as Sativex, is another prescription cannabinoid product and was the first approved medicine to be completely derived from *C. sativa*. It is an almost 1:1 ratio of plant extractions of THC and CBD and is approved for pain associated with either spasticity or neuropathic pain related to multiple sclerosis (MS). In Canada and Israel Sativex is approved for use to treat cancer pain in patients unresponsive to opiates. In the USA, Sativex was studied as a treatment for cancer pain but failed phase III clinical trials and was not approved. Epidiolex, a CBD completely extracted from the cannabis plant, was recently approved first in the USA and shortly after by the EU. In both the USA and EU, Epidiolex was approved for the adjunctive treatment of two childhood epilepsies, Lennox–Gastaut syndrome (LGS) and Dravet syndrome (DS). In addition to LGS and DS, Epidiolex is also approved in the EU for the indication of seizures related to tuberous sclerosis.

Table 4.1 Prescription cannabinoids

	Nabiximols (Sativex)	Cannabidiol (Epidiolex)	Dronabinol (Marinol)	Dronabinol (Syndros)	Nabilone (Cesamet)
Description	Combination THC + CBD extracts from approved C. *sativa* cultivars	CBD extract from approved C. *sativa* cultivars	Synthetic THC in sesame-oil gel	Synthetic THC in liquid solution	Modified synthetic THC
Approved	UK, Canada, some EU	USA, UK, EU	USA, Canada, UK, some EU, Australia, New Zealand	USA only	USA, Canada, UK, some EU including Germany and Spain
Indications (may be different between countries)	Spasticity in MS	Lennox–Gastaut syndrome Dravet syndrome Seizures associated with tuberous sclerosis (EU)	CINV Anorexia with HIV	CINV Anorexia with HIV	CINV Anorexia with HIV Spasticity in MS Chronic pain glaucoma

CBD, cannabidiol; CINV, chemotherapy-induced nausea and vomiting; MS, multiple sclerosis; THC, Δ^9-tetrahydrocannabinol.

During this period from 1985 to the present, as regulatory authorities approved these cannabinoid-based prescription medicines, in many of these countries access to the phyto-cannabinoids found in marijuana was liberalized and criminal penalties reconsidered. In an increasing number of countries marijuana is now available for medical use (termed medical marijuana) and in Canada, Uruguay and an increasing number of states within the USA for recreational use as well. This increased access to marijuana has been driven by several factors including growing social acceptance, a change in governmental policies that reflect the belief that prohibition of use and criminal penalties were too severe, and a belief that cannabis use is safe. Although these changes will continue to evolve, it is important to keep in mind that these perceptions are often driven by social and political factors. Scientific evidence still lags behind and awaits future investment in research.

Over time more information about medical marijuana and recreational use of marijuana will inevitably be collected and the benefits and risks of patient exposure will be better understood. Unlike prescription drugs, marijuana is not an approved product and no formalized program to systematically collect information on efficacy, safety and adverse events is available. Although occasional use may appear not to pose serious concerns, the safety of increased potency of cannabis from higher concentrations of THC and the longer exposure when used for chronic medical conditions or simply increased social acceptance has yet to be determined. With this increased exposure, cannabis dependence, addiction and withdrawal symptoms have been increasingly recognized as public health challenges with the highest incidence in the world found in the USA at 148 users per 1000 adults. In Europe, the rates are lower with the highest rate in Spain at 96 per 1000 followed by the Czech Republic at 92 per 1000 and France 84 per 1000 (United Nations Office on Drugs and Crime, 2014). Overall, cannabis use worldwide is estimated at nearly 200 million.

Although more information is needed to better determine how cannabinoids as a class are used or abused, reports in peer-reviewed scientific literature can provide help. One highly respected and widely used publication is the *Cochrane Database of Systematic Reviews*. This includes Cochrane Reviews, which are comprehensive reviews of the medical literature on selected topics, and is completely independent of any commercial influence. Six Cochrane Reviews have been published in recent years that review cannabinoids used as potential therapeutic agents. Topics reported have included CINV (Smith and Jess, 2011), anorexia and HIV (Lutge, Gray and Siegfried, 2013), epilepsy (Gloss and Vickrey, 2011), fibromyalgia (Walitt *et al.*, 2016), cannabis dependence (Marshall, Gowing and Ali, 2011) and schizophrenia (McLoughlin *et al.*, 2014).

In addition to these comprehensive reviews, two non-Cochrane medical literature reviews have been published recently. The first of these was conducted by the American Academy of Neurology (AAN) and surveyed published data from 1948 to November 2013 of RCTs of cannabinoids in several preselected disease states. Since the first synthetic cannabinoid was unavailable before 1985, the first 37 years only report the results of the use of phytocannabinoids including marijuana. The AAN review selected the areas of MS, epilepsy and movement disorders. Their search identified 34 studies that were deemed of sufficient size and quality to be included and 8 were considered as Class I (high-quality) studies.

The authors concluded that in MS, oral cannabis extracts (OCE) were effective with nabiximols (Sativex) and THC probably effective in reduction of patient-centered measures of pain during the clinical study and possibly patient-centered and objective measures of pain continued after one year. OCE was also effective for central pain and painful spasms excluding neuropathic pain with both nabiximols and THC probably effective. Nabiximols was also regarded as probably effective for urinary complaints in MS while OCE and THC were ineffective. None of the agents (OCE, THC, dronabinol and nabiximols) were useful in relieving tremor related to MS.

The authors also concluded that there was inadequate evidence to determine the efficacy of cannabinoids in movement disorders or epilepsy due to insufficient clinical data to review (Koppel *et al.*, 2014). It should be remembered that this review was published several years before the approval of Epidiolex, a CBD now available as adjunctive treatment for several rare pediatric epilepsies.

A second independent survey was published shortly after the AAN paper in the *Journal of the American Medical Association* (JAMA). In this review, the authors pooled data from published studies and compared cannabinoids (phytocannabinoids and approved chemically synthetic cannabinoids) with standard of care, placebo or no treatment over the preceding 40 years of published RCTs that enrolled more than 25 patients. Ten clinical disorders were identified within this meta-analysis for study (Whiting *et al.*, 2015) and despite the limitations inherent with meta-analysis, the study concluded moderate evidence was available in published studies to support the use of cannabinoids for spasticity and chronic pain. Although dronabinol and nabilone were FDA approved for CINV and anorexia associated with HIV, overall the authors believed only low-quality evidence of benefit was found for these conditions and also for weight gain, sleep disorders and Tourette's syndrome. No evidence of benefit was found for the treatment of depression but only three studies were identified in the analysis (Whiting *et al.*, 2015). In Chapter 7 we will review later studies on cannabinoids and depression.

Nabilone (Cesamet)

After THC was isolated from *C. sativa* and subsequently made from a chemical synthesis, efforts to chemically modify the molecule and develop new medicines quickly followed. Nabilone was synthesized in 1975 and later became the first synthetic analog of THC approved for clinical use. Through a simple chemical substitution of a ketone group for a methyl group on one of the three rings of THC, nabilone retained the affinity to bind as a partial agonist to both the CB_1 and CB_2 receptors. This small change in structure, however, significantly altered the degradation of nabilone. One consequence of this molecular reengineering was a significant difference in the hepatic metabolism and metabolites produced (Lemberger and Rowe, 1975). This allowed nabilone to retain important properties as a cannabinoid receptor agonist while differentiating itself in unique pharmacokinetic and pharmacodynamic characteristics.

Nabilone is available as a hard gelatin capsule and rapidly absorbed from the intestinal tract. The medication is highly bioavailable (96%) with a half-life of approximately 2 hours. Nabilone is subjected to extensive metabolism but does not undergo the carboxylation process that occurs with THC. The absence of a carboxylate metabolite results in nabilone being undetectable in blood and urine using the standard assays for cannabinoids. The molecule is instead broken down into a number of isomeric alcohols and eliminated primarily through the fecal route (65%) with less urinary excretion (20%) (Ward and Holmes, 1985).

Early animal studies revealed that nabilone had antiemetic properties similar to THC and eventually led to clinical trials as a treatment for CINV (Ware, Daeninck and Maida,

2008). In 1986 nabilone was approved for CINV in the UK but approval in the USA was delayed for commercial reasons until 2006. Follow-up studies continued to confirm the antiemetic properties of nabilone although the use of the drug was limited as a result of troubling side effects that included postural hypotension, dizziness, drowsiness and tachycardia (Tramèr et al., 2001). With the introduction beginning in the 1990s of other classes of antiemetics including the 5-HT_{3A} and NK_1 receptor antagonists that were better tolerated, nabilone became a second-line treatment in CINV and today has only limited use (Ware, Daeninck and Maida, 2008).

Although CINV remains the most frequent use for nabilone prescriptions, clinical studies have explored novel uses for the drug including neuropathic pain and fibromyalgia (Skrabek et al., 2008). Ware et al. (2010) in a two-week, randomized, double-blind study of 29 patients that compared nabilone with the low-dose tricyclic amitriptyline in fibromyalgia and severe insomnia reported no change in pain or mood although sleep was improved with both conditions. Compared with amitriptyline, nabilone was better at achieving the primary outcome of improved sleep quality (Ware et al., 2010).

There have been other studies of nabilone that have also failed to demonstrate analgesic benefits in pain syndromes. Guindon and Beaulieu (2006) evaluated nabilone in an acute pain model of 41 patients undergoing surgical procedures. Patients were treated postoperatively with nabilone, ketoprofen or placebo for 24 hours after the procedure. Pain was considerably worse with nabilone than ketoprofen and in fact nabilone did little better than placebo (Guindon and Beaulieu, 2006). In another pain study nabilone was studied in chronic neuropathic pain and reported to be inferior to hydrocodone (Frank et al., 2008). However, when evaluated as an adjunctive analgesic in a crossover design in chronic pain, nabilone was reported to be beneficial as an add-on medication (Pinsger et al., 2006).

Early preclinical studies also indicated that nabilone might be useful as an anxiolytic and antipsychotic medication (Lemberger and Rowe, 1975). In a placebo-controlled study of 25 patients with anxiety, nabilone showed significant reduction of anxiety although side effects limited the potential usefulness and acceptance by the patients of the drug (Fabre and McLendon, 1981). Much later, a retrospective case study of 47 combat veterans diagnosed with post-traumatic stress disorder (PTSD) reported a significant reduction in the frequency and intensity of nightmares with an improvement in quality of sleep with nabilone (Fraser, 2009). Nabilone has also been investigated in cannabis dependence as an agonist replacement treatment. However, in a randomized, placebo-controlled clinical trial of 18 patients with DSM-IV diagnosis of cannabis abuse, no statistical difference was found in patient self-report between nabilone and placebo (Hill et al., 2017).

Dronabinol (Marinol and Syndros)

Unlike nabilone, dronabinol is not an analog of the THC molecule. Instead, dronabinol is the identical molecular structure of THC although it is made through a chemical synthesis rather than as an extraction from C. sativa. Dronabinol was first approved in 1985 for CINV in the USA as a soft gel capsule and in 2016 as a liquid formulation given orally and dissolved in ethanol. As a product of chemical synthesis, dronabinol is a pure THC formulation without the contaminants and impurities of extraction from a botanical source. In contrast to nabilone, since dronabinol is the molecular twin of THC, the general pharmacokinetics and metabolic degradation are identical to THC. THC is typically delivered by smoking or ingestion while dronabinol is provided as a gel capsule or oral solution.

These differences in delivery account for variations in how the drug is absorbed by the body when compared with THC. In addition, the prescription dronabinol avoids the considerable hazards of smoked THC.

The development of dronabinol as a prescription medication has had an unusual journey through the drug regulatory process. Prior to the introduction of dronabinol as an approved pharmaceutical drug, there was a growing awareness among scientists and the public of the potential health benefits of cannabis. Marijuana was the first drug allowed in the USA to bypass the FDA approval process required of all prescription drugs and be used for compassionate treatment. In the 1970s, an individual with glaucoma refractory to available medications at that time was allowed to legally smoke marijuana to alleviate his symptoms. This is discussed in greater detail in Chapter 10 in the glaucoma description. At the same time, the antiemetic effects of marijuana were also becoming recognized and offered significant relief from nausea and vomiting in patients undergoing poorly tolerated chemotherapy (Sallan *et al.*, 1980). These reports of the therapeutic benefits of smoked marijuana placed the political and regulatory authorities in a difficult situation by requiring the US government to provide marijuana to patients for compassionate use while criminalizing the possession or use of cannabis. The development of a pure, synthetic THC that could be regulated and safety monitored through established drug safety programs offered an alternative (and legal) way to treat refractory disorders without the government obligated to grow and distribute marijuana.

To develop and then commercialize dronabinol, however, was a daunting task that few pharmaceutical companies desired to pursue. Because THC was an illegal substance as a Schedule I drug, access to drug supply for clinical trials would be a difficult and long experience and there was an uncertain feeling that it would ever be approved for human use with no guarantee of clinical or commercial success. To overcome these obstacles, the US government provided the vast majority of the funding to Unimed, a small pharmaceutical company that by itself did not have the resources to develop dronabinol. In addition, because of the medical need the FDA agreed to accelerate the approval process. The typical time for a successful drug development is usually several years but for dronabinol the timeline was compressed to two years.

In 1985 dronabinol was approved in the USA under the brand name Marinol for CINV. This was followed several years later by the approval for a second indication, anorexia associated with HIV. Similar to the earlier exceptions with the approval of dronabinol for CINV, the authorization for anorexia associated with HIV received considerable government support due to the growing AIDS crisis and the absence of available treatments. Dronabinol was approved in 1992 for wasting related to anorexia in HIV.

In 2016 a second dronabinol product, Syndros, was approved for the identical indications as Marinol. Both products are synthetic THC but differ in the delivery of dronabinol. Marinol is dronabinol in a soft gel capsule available as 2.5 mg, 5 mg and 10 mg capsules. Syndros, named because it is synthetic dronabinol in oral solution, is dronabinol in solution with ethanol mixed with water when administered. Although Marinol was rescheduled to Schedule III, Syndros remains in Schedule II as a result of the use of ethanol in the formulation. Syndros is dosed using a dosing guideline similar to guidelines used in determining the dose in chemotherapy. Syndros is dosed for CINV on the basis of body surface area at 4.2 mg/m^2 from 1 to 2 hours before chemotherapy is administered. Repeated doses at 2–4 hours up to 4–6 times a day are allowed for the administration of Syndros and can be provided throughout the course of chemotherapy. Food can delay the absorption of

Syndros, and administration is recommended on an empty stomach at least 30 minutes before meals. For induction of appetite in HIV patients with wasting, the dosage is different and much simpler and starts at 2.1 mg orally twice daily and titrated up to 4.2 mg twice daily (Syndros PI).

Both Marinol and Syndros are pharmaceutical pure products of THC produced through chemical synthesis. No botanical extractions from *C. sativa* are involved in the process and impurities that are usually associated with botanical extractions are absent.

In understanding how THC and the synthetic dronabinol and nabilone work, preclinical studies have provided insight into the role of the endocannabinoid system (ECS) in the control of nausea and vomiting. It is now well established that CB_1 and CB_2 receptors in the brain stem are involved in the regulation of emesis (Hornby, 2001; Van Sickle *et al.*, 2005). In preclinical work, the endocannabinoid 2-arachidonoylglycerol (2-AG) has been found to be elevated in the insular cortex of rodents (Sticht *et al.*, 2016) during episodes of nausea. Inhibition of the ECS degradation systems, namely fatty acid amide hydrolase (FAAH) and monoacylglycerol lipase (MAGL), and elevation of the endocannabinoids have been reported to reduce nausea in rodent studies. As described in Chapters 2 and 3, THC and the endocannabinoids act on many receptors other than the cannabinoid receptors. THC is known to act at the $5\text{-}HT_3$ receptor and cannabinoids likely act through both the cannabinoid receptors in the ECS and through other receptors including $5\text{-}HT_3$ in the modulation of nausea and vomiting (Barann *et al.*, 2002).

Several clinical studies in humans have confirmed the effects of dronabinol in the treatment of CINV. In one meta-analysis of RCTs enrolling more than 25 patients, 28 studies on CINV were identified and included 1772 participants treated with either dronabinol, nabilone or THC (Whiting *et al.*, 2015). Meta-analysis can often provide interesting insights into the variety of treatments patients receive but can also be inconclusive due to the pooling of many studies of varying design and quality. In a study reported by Meiri *et al.* (2007), the authors concluded only low-quality evidence existed that cannabinoid medicines relieved CINV. Three studies were included in the analysis and only one evaluated dronabinol as monotherapy. The other two dronabinol studies reviewed the use of the drug as an add-on medication with either ondansetron or prochlorperazine. Only in a small study was dronabinol reported to be equivalent to ondansetron in the treatment of CINV. When used as an add-on medication to this $5\text{-}HT_3$ antagonist, no additional benefit was found (Meiri *et al.*, 2007). Although both nabilone and dronabinol are approved to be effective in treating CINV, the more recent $5\text{-}HT_3$ and NK_1 antagonists are better tolerated and much preferred by patients.

Nabiximols (Sativex)

Nabiximols is a cannabinoid plant extract that contains a combination of THC (27 mg/ml) plus CBD (25 mg/ml) administered as an oromucosal spray. Unlike nabilone and dronabinol that are synthesized from chemical processes, nabiximols is extracted from the cannabis plant under rigorous growing conditions and, in addition to THC and CBD, contains minor impurities and contaminants considered acceptable by various regulatory agencies including the European Medicines Agency (EMA) and Health Canada. Although not as pure as synthetic cannabinoids, nabiximols had to establish an adequate level of purity of THC and CBD to be approved as a pharmaceutical product and is monitored by the regulatory authorities as for all approved medications for continuing efficacy and safety. Although nabiximols has been approved in over 30 countries including Canada, the UK and others in the EU, it is not available in the USA. Recently nabiximols failed three late-stage clinical trials for cancer pain and was not approved by the FDA and any future development in the USA is unknown.

Nabiximols is approved in 30 countries for use as an adjunctive treatment for pain and spasticity in MS. In Canada and Israel nabiximols is also approved for neuropathic pain in MS and a second indication for pain in advanced cancer uncontrolled by opiates.

Earlier isolated studies with cannabis reported in the 1980s and 1990s suggested benefits in reducing spasticity in MS (Brenneisen *et al.*, 1996). Several large, well-controlled, randomized studies followed and included nabiximols with promising findings (Wade *et al.*, 2004, 2010). Patients with MS present with diverse symptoms and disabilities impacted by the disease and were questioned about the most troubling symptom out of five common complaints: spasticity, pain, bladder dysfunction, tremor or spasms. In those patients that identified spasticity as the most troublesome complaint, nabiximols showed the most significant improvement when compared with placebo. Treatment with nabiximols showed only minimal benefit on the other four symptoms. Several RCTs have since followed and continue to report the efficacy of nabiximols as an adjunctive treatment to relieve spasticity associated with MS (Novotna *et al.*, 2011).

Despite these studies, the usefulness of nabiximols remains in question. For example, the Ashworth Scale is a validated and objective clinician assessment frequently used in spasticity studies and nabiximols studies in spasticity using the Ashworth Scale as the primary outcome have been inconsistent. Other assessments commonly used in spasticity studies include the numeric rating scale (NRS), visual analog scale (VAS) and patient reported outcomes (PRO). These scales have been more consistent in demonstrating benefit for patients treated with nabiximols (Farrar *et al.*, 2008) and some have suggested that these subjective measures may be more relevant in the overall patient complaints with spasticity (Fleuren *et al.*, 2010).

As mentioned earlier, neuropathic pain associated with MS is another approved indication for nabiximols as an adjunctive treatment. Nurmikko *et al.* (2007) studied 125 patients with neuropathic pain of peripheral origin in a five-week, randomized, double-blind, placebo-controlled, parallel design trial. Pain intensity scores were the primary outcome in the study and 63 patients received nabiximols and the remaining 62 received placebo. Patients on nabiximols were found to have a greater reduction in pain scores compared with placebo. Secondary outcomes all were found to favor nabiximols over placebo including a NRS, Neuropathic Pain Scale composite score, sleep, dynamic allodynia and punctate allodynia and Pain Disability Index (PDI). Following the clinical trial patients were allowed to continue in a 52-week, open-label extension study. In the continuation study patients continued to maintain their initial pain relief without dose escalation or toxicity for 52 weeks (Nurmikko *et al.*, 2007).

In another study of neuropathic pain Berman *et al.* (2004) evaluated 48 patients with pain and allodynia and at least one avulsed root in a randomized, double-blind, placebo-controlled, three-period crossover study. After a two-week baseline, three two-week treatment periods followed during which patients received either one of two oromucosal spray preparations of nabiximols or a placebo. The primary outcome measure was the mean pain severity score collected during the final seven days of treatment (Berman, Symonds and Birch, 2004).

Cannabidiol (CBD) (Epidiolex)

Epidiolex is the most recent cannabinoid-based medication approved and is extracted CBD from the cannabis plant. It is available as an oral solution of 100 mg/ml and recommended to be given initially at 2.5 mg/kg twice daily. After one week the dosage can be increased to a maintenance dosage of 5 mg/kg twice daily.

In 2018 the FDA granted approval for Epidiolex in the USA for the treatment of two treatment-resistant epilepsies in childhood. Epidiolex is now available by prescription for DS and LGS in the USA and in the EU a third indication of seizures related to tuberous sclerosis has been added. Three large clinical trials were completed that evaluated Epidiolex as an adjunctive treatment for these devastating seizure disorders of childhood. Over 560 patients were studied in randomized, placebo-controlled, double-blind studies with significant reductions in seizure numbers reported.

The first published study that CBD might be effective for treatment-resistant epilepsy was a study of adult and pediatric patients with refractory seizures at 11 epilepsy centers in the USA. All patients had previously failed conventional treatments and the dosage of Epidiolex began at 2.5 mg/kg per day and could be titrated up to a maximum of 25–50 mg/kg per day. The median decrease in total seizures in the 130 patients studied in this expanded access program was 34.6% (Devinsky et al., 2016). Several large-scale studies followed this report and in a pooled analysis of 580 patients the median monthly frequency of seizures was reduced by 51% and the frequency of total seizures by 48% (Gaston and Szaflarski, 2018; Szaflarski et al., 2018).

Three additional studies followed, and all were conducted in a double-blind, placebo-controlled trial design with a 4-week baseline followed by 2 weeks of dosage titration and 12 weeks of combination therapy. The patients were tapered off medication over 10 days and then followed with a four-week safety assessment. The primary outcome in all three studies was a percentage change in the primary seizure with multiple secondary measurements that included the reduction of seizures other than the primary seizure and caregiver impression of change (CGIC).

In the first study, 61 adult and pediatric patients with DS were treated with median seizure frequency reduction of 38.9%. Three patients were seizure free and 62% of the caregivers reported improvement of CBD compared with the placebo (Devinsky et al., 2017).

The second study randomized 171 adult and pediatric patients diagnosed with LGS. Similar to the first study with DS patients, the primary outcome of monthly seizure frequency decreased in the CBD group compared with the placebo by 43.9% to 21.8%. In patients treated with CBD, 44% of them demonstrated at least a 50% reduction. CGIC was also significant with 58% improved on CBD (Thiele et al., 2018).

In the final study 225 adult and pediatric patients with LGS were randomized and two doses (10 mg/kg per day and 20 mg/kg per day) of CBD were compared with placebo. Both doses of CBD demonstrated significant efficacy compared with placebo. The primary outcome was monthly seizure frequency which decreased by 41% at a dose of 20 mg/kg per day and by 37.2% with the lower dose of 10 mg/kg per day. Placebo response in the study was 17.2% reduction from the baseline (Devinsky et al., 2018).

Side effects reported in the open-label expanded access program and the three RCTs were very similar. Diarrhea (29.2%) and somnolence (22.4%) were the most common reported adverse events and are consistent with the side effects noted in the use of cannabinoids (Gaston and Szaflarski, 2018). Elevations in liver function tests occurred in 10% of patients on CBD with the majority of this group also commonly treated without valproate and clobazam.

As discussed earlier in Chapter 2, THC and CBD are primarily metabolized through the CYP3A4 and CYP2C19 isoenzymes in the liver. These well-controlled trials of CBD in LGS and DS provide additional high-quality information regarding the hepatic metabolism. Since Epidiolex is prescribed as an adjunctive to other medications that can affect the liver, appropriate care should be exercised when known inducers or inhibitors of these metabolic pathways are coadministered with CBD.

Conversations to Have with Patients

The cannabinoid-based medicines nabilone and dronabinol were first approved for the treatment of CINV. This was followed several years later with a second approval for dronabinol to treat anorexia associated with HIV. Substantial regulatory and legal barriers had to be overcome in the development of these medications since marijuana was an illegal substance and access to the psychoactive THC was highly restricted. Only the fact that THC could address several urgent unmet medical needs allowed the studies to be conducted.

Today, neither dronabinol nor nabilone are widely used for either indication. For emesis, new classes of medications have emerged that are equally effective and much better tolerated. Nausea is less well managed with the newer medicines, however, and future development of drugs that enhance the availability of endocannabinoids potentially could provide alternative treatments of nausea.

Similarly, for appetite stimulation of anorexia associated with HIV patients, dronabinol has had only a limited success. Advances in the treatment of HIV and the poor tolerability of dronabinol in many patients has limited the use of this medicine to treat appetite reduction.

Despite being able to have access to THC in dronabinol or nabilone as a legal prescription, many patients prefer to smoke marijuana even in instances when it has been illegal. There are several reasons that may account for this behavior. One may be the rapid uptake of cannabis through smoking compared with the delayed absorption of oral consumption. The ability to have an effect rapidly through inhalation and to easily titrate dosage would be difficult for any product absorbed in the intestinal tract. However, there is another factor that may be even more challenging for prescription cannabinoid-based medicines to overcome. As discussed in Chapter 1, cannabis is a mixture of many phytocannabinoids including THC and CBD plus terpenes and flavonoids. The mixture of several hundred different potentially biologically active molecules creates what is known as the entourage effect (Ben-Shabat *et al.*, 1998). The entourage effect is a synergistic effect of many molecular elements within cannabis and may vary based upon the cultivar of the plant and environmental variation. Frequently patients can better tolerate (and prefer) the mixed entourage ingredients of cannabis rather than one purified molecule from a chemical synthesis in the laboratory. Demonstrating superiority in efficacy and better tolerability and safety will be difficult challenges for drug development to overcome.

Nabiximols was the first drug approved that consisted of botanical extraction of constituents from the cannabis plant. As a totally derived, plant-based product, nabiximols consists of approximately a 1:1 ratio of THC and CBD plus minor contaminants of other cannabinoids and terpenes produced in the plant. It has been approved in more countries worldwide for more indications than any other prescription cannabinoid. This cannabinoid combination from *C. sativa* appears to be well tolerated but the comparisons of nabiximols with smoked cannabis have yet to be published.

Epidiolex is CBD, the second botanical extraction from *C. sativa,* and was approved with much anticipation in the USA and EU for the treatment of resistant pediatric seizures. CBD may have many more uses in the future beyond epilepsy, but considerable investment and effort must occur before new indications for use can occur. In the meantime, CBD preparations as herbs and topicals are available and heavily promoted with claims yet to be proven.

Determining whether products developed through the formal drug approval process are better than "medical marijuana" will be a critical issue in the near future. Recently in a meta-analysis of seizures by Pamplona *et al.* (2018) that compared CBD-rich extracts with the more purified CBD in Epidiolex, both treatments appeared equally effective in reducing seizures. However, the total CBD in the CBD-enriched extracts was found to be one-fourth the dosage of the more purified CBD raising multiple questions on dosage and safety (Pamplona, Da Silva and Coan, 2018).

Future studies will need to address these questions. Only when clinical trials and observational studies are completed will we know if further innovation will occur.

Bibliography

Barann, M. *et al.* (2002) 'Direct inhibition by cannabinoids of human 5-HT 3A receptors: probable involvement of an allosteric modulatory site', *British Journal of Pharmacology*, 137(5), 589–596. doi:10.1038/sj.bjp.0704829.

Ben-Shabat, S. *et al.* (1998) 'An entourage effect: inactive endogenous fatty acid glycerol esters enhance 2-arachidonoyl-glycerol cannabinoid activity', *European Journal of Pharmacology*, 353(1), 23–31. doi:10.1016/S0014-2999(98)00392-6.

Berman, J. S., Symonds, C. and Birch, R. (2004) 'Efficacy of two cannabis based medicinal extracts for relief of central neuropathic pain from brachial plexus avulsion: results of a randomised controlled trial', *Pain*, 112(3), 299–306. doi:10.1016/j.pain.2004.09.013.

Brenneisen, R. *et al.* (1996) 'The effect of orally and rectally administered delta 9-tetrahydrocannabinol on spasticity: a pilot study with 2 patients.', *International Journal of Clinical Pharmacology and Therapeutics*, 34 (10), 446–452. Available at: www.ncbi.nlm.nih.gov/pubmed/8897084.

Devinsky, O. *et al.* (2016) 'Cannabidiol in patients with treatment-resistant epilepsy: an open-label interventional trial', *The Lancet Neurology*, 15(3), 270–278. doi:10.1016/S1474-4422(15)00379-8.

Devinsky, O. *et al.* (2017) 'Trial of cannabidiol for drug-resistant seizures in the Dravet syndrome', *New England Journal of Medicine*, 376(21), 2011–2020. doi:10.1056/NEJMoa1611618.

Devinsky, O. *et al.* (2018) 'Effect of cannabidiol on drop seizures in the Lennox-Gastaut syndrome', *New England Journal of Medicine*, 378, 1888–1897.

Fabre, L. F. and McLendon, D. (1981) 'The efficacy and safety of nabilone (a synthetic cannabinoid) in the treatment of anxiety', *The Journal of Clinical Pharmacology*, 21(S1), 377S-382S. doi:10.1002/j.1552-4604.1981.tb02617.x.

Farrar, J. T. *et al.* (2008) 'Validity, reliability, and clinical importance of change in a 0–10 numeric rating scale measure of spasticity: a post hoc analysis of a randomized, double-blind, placebo-controlled trial', *Clinical Therapeutics*, 30(5), 974–985. doi:10.1016/j.clinthera.2008.05.011.

Fleuren, J. F. M. *et al.* (2010) 'Stop using the Ashworth Scale for the assessment of spasticity', *Journal of Neurology, Neurosurgery and Psychiatry*, 81(1), 46–52. doi:10.1136/jnnp.2009.177071.

Frank, B. *et al.* (2008) 'Comparison of analgesic effects and patient tolerability of nabilone and dihydrocodeine for chronic neuropathic pain: randomised, crossover, double blind study', *BMJ*, 336(7637), 199–201. doi:10.1136/bmj.39429.619653.80.

Fraser, G. A. (2009) 'The use of a synthetic cannabinoid in the management of treatment-resistant nightmares in posttraumatic stress disorder (PTSD)', *CNS Neuroscience and Therapeutics*, 15(1), 84–88. doi:10.1111/j.1755-5949.2008.00071.x.

Gaston, T. E. and Szaflarski, J. P. (2018) 'Cannabis for the treatment of epilepsy: an update', *Current Neurology and Neuroscience Reports*, 18(11), 1–9. doi:10.1007/s11910-018-0882-y.

Gloss, D. and Vickrey, B. (2011) 'Cannabinoids for epilepsy', *Cochrane Database of Systematic Reviews*, 3, CD009270. doi:10.1002/14651858.CD009270.pub3.

Guindon, J. and Beaulieu, P. (2006) 'Antihyperalgesic effects of local injections of anandamide, ibuprofen, rofecoxib and their combinations in a model of neuropathic pain', *Neuropharmacology*, 50(7), 814–823. doi:10.1016/j.neuropharm.2005.12.002.

Hill, K. P. *et al.* (2017) 'Nabilone pharmacotherapy for cannabis dependence: a randomized, controlled pilot study', *The American Journal on Addictions*, 26(8), 795–801. doi:10.1111/ajad.12622.

Hornby, P. J. (2001) 'Central neurocircuitry associated with emesis', *American Journal of Medicine*, 111(8 Suppl 1), 106–112. doi:10.1016/s0002-9343(01)00849-x.

Koppel, B. S. *et al.* (2014) 'Systematic review: efficacy and safety of medical marijuana in selected neurologic disorders: Report of the Guideline Development Subcommittee of the American Academy of Neurology', *Neurology*, 82(17), 1556–1563. doi:10.1212/WNL.0000000000000363.

Lemberger, L. and Rowe, H. (1975) 'Clinical pharmacology of nabilone, a cannabinol derivative', *Clinical Pharmacology & Therapeutics*, 18(6), 720–726. doi:10.1002/cpt1975186720.

Lutge, E. E., Gray, A. and Siegfried, N. (2013) 'The medical use of cannabis for reducing morbidity and mortality in patients with HIV/ AIDS', *Cochrane Database of Systematic Reviews*, 4, CD005175. doi:10.1002/14651858.CD005175.pub3.

Marshall, K. S., Gowing, L. and Ali, R. (2011) 'Pharmacotherapies for cannabis withdrawal', *Cochrane Database of Systematic Reviews*, 1, CD008940. doi:10.1002/14651858.CD008940.

McLoughlin, B. C. *et al.* (2014) 'Cannabis and schizophrenia', *Cochrane Database of Systematic Reviews*, 10, CD004837. doi:10.1002/14651858.CD004837.pub3.

Meiri, E. *et al.* (2007) 'Efficacy of dronabinol alone and in combination with ondansetron versus ondansetron alone for delayed chemotherapy-induced nausea and vomiting', *Current Medical Research and Opinion*, 23(3), 533–543. doi:10.1185/030079907X167525.

Novotna, A. *et al.* (2011) 'A randomized, double-blind, placebo-controlled, parallel-group, enriched-design study of nabiximols* (Sativex ®), as add-on therapy, in subjects with refractory spasticity caused by multiple sclerosis', *European Journal of Neurology*, 18 (9), 1122–1131. doi:10.1111/j.1468-1331.2010.03328.x.

Nurmikko, T. J. *et al.* (2007) 'Sativex successfully treats neuropathic pain characterised by allodynia: a randomised, double-blind, placebo-controlled clinical trial', *Pain*, 133 (1–3), 210–220. doi:10.1016/j.pain.2007.08.028.

Pamplona, F. A., Da Silva, L. R. and Coan, A. C. (2018) 'Potential clinical benefits of CBD-rich cannabis extracts over purified CBD in treatment-resistant epilepsy: observational data meta-analysis', *Frontiers in Neurology*, 9, 759. doi:10.3389/fneur.2018.00759.

Pinsger, M. *et al.* (2006) 'Nutzen einer add-on-therapie mit dem synthetischen cannabinomimetikum nabilone bei patienten mit chronischen schmerzzuständen – Eine randomisierte kontrollierte studie', *Wiener Klinische Wochenschrift*, 118(11–12), 327–335. doi:10.1007/s00508-006-0611-4.

Sallan, S. E. *et al.* (1980) 'Antiemetics in patients receiving chemotherapy for cancer — a randomized comparison of delta-9-tetrahydrocannabinol and prochlorperazine', *New England Journal of Medicine*, 302, 135–138. doi:10.1056/NEJM198001173020302.

Skrabek, R. Q. *et al.* (2008) 'Nabilone for the treatment of pain in fibromyalgia', *The Journal of Pain*, 9(2), 164–173. doi:10.1016/j.jpain.2007.09.002.

Smith, L. A. and Jess, C. E. (2011) 'Cannabinoids for nausea and vomiting in cancer patients receiving chemotherapy', *Cochrane Database of Systematic Reviews*, 11, CD009464. doi:10.1002/14651858.CD009464.

Sticht, M. A. *et al.* (2016) 'Endocannabinoid regulation of nausea is mediated by 2-arachidonoylglycerol (2-AG) in the rat visceral insular cortex', *Neuropharmacology*, 102, 92–102. doi:10.1016/j.neuropharm.2015.10.039.

Szaflarski, J. P. *et al.* (2018) 'Long-term safety and treatment effects of cannabidiol in children and adults with treatment-resistant epilepsies: expanded access program results', *Epilepsia*, 59(8), 1540–1548. doi:10.1111/epi.14477.

Thiele, E. A. *et al.* (2018) 'Cannabidiol in patients with seizures associated with Lennox-Gastaut syndrome (GWPCARE4): a randomised, double-blind, placebo-controlled phase 3 trial', *The Lancet*, 391(10125), 1085–1096. doi:10.1016/S0140-6736(18)30136-3.

Tramèr, M. R. *et al.* (2001) 'Cannabinoids for control of chemotherapy induced nausea and vomiting: quantitative systematic review', *British Medical Journal*, 323(7303), 16–21.

United Nations Office on Drugs and Crime (2014) *World Drug Report 2014* (United Nations publication, Sales No. E.14.XI.7).

Van Sickle, M. D. *et al.* (2005) 'Neuroscience: identification and functional characterization of brainstem cannabinoid CB$_2$ receptors', *Science*, 310(5746), 329–332. doi:10.1126/science.1115740.

Wade, D. T. *et al.* (2004) 'Do cannabis-based medicinal extracts have general or specific effects on symptoms in multiple sclerosis? A double-blind, randomized, placebo-controlled study on 160 patients', *Multiple Sclerosis Journal*, 10(4), 434–441. doi:10.1191/1352458504ms1082oa.

Wade, D. T. *et al.* (2010) 'Meta-analysis of the efficacy and safety of Sativex (nabiximols), on spasticity in people with multiple sclerosis', *Multiple Sclerosis Journal*, 16(6), 707–714. doi:10.1177/1352458510367462.

Walitt, B. *et al.* (2016) 'Cannabinoids for fibromyalgia', *Cochrane Database of Systematic Reviews*, 7, CD011694. doi:10.1002/14651858.CD011694.pub2.

Ward, A. and Holmes, B. (1985) 'Nabilone: a preliminary review of its pharmacological properties and therapeutic use', *Drugs*, 30(2), 127–144. doi:10.2165/00003495-198530020-00002.

Ware, M. A. *et al.* (2010) 'The effects of nabilone on sleep in fibromyalgia: results of a randomized controlled trial', *Anesthesia and Analgesia*, 110(2), 604–610. doi:10.1213/ANE.0b013e3181c76f70.

Ware, M. A., Daeninck, P. and Maida, V. (2008) 'A review of nabilone in the treatment of chemotherapy-induced nausea and vomiting', *Therapeutics and Clinical Risk Management*, 4(1), 99–107. doi:10.2147/tcrm.s1132.

Whiting, P. F. *et al.* (2015) 'Cannabinoids for medical use: a systematic review and meta-analysis', *JAMA: Journal of the American Medical Association*, 313(24), 2456–2473. doi:10.1001/jama.2015.6358.

The Safety of Phytocannabinoids and Cannabinoids in Clinical Practice

Doctors put drugs of which they know little into bodies of which they know less for diseases they know nothing at all.

Voltaire

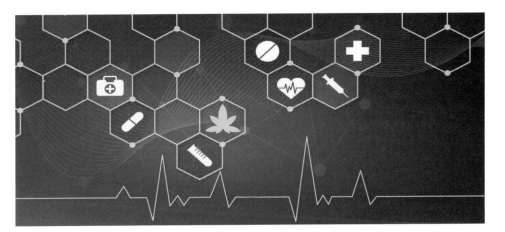

- Medical marijuana is not approved for use by any regulatory authority worldwide.
- Cannabis use and concentration of Δ^9-tetrahydrocannabinol (THC) has increased with smoked and vaporized marijuana the two most preferred methods.
- Several acute and chronic pulmonary effects are associated with smoking or vaping including inflammation of the airways and damage to lung parenchyma.
- Cannabis use is associated with a threefold increase of inducing manic symptoms in bipolar disorder. There appears to be a dose-dependent effect on the precipitation of psychosis in predisposed individuals and an earlier occurrence of illness in cannabis users.
- Cannabis use disorder has become a well-recognized and accepted condition and is defined both in DSM-5 and ICD-10 criteria.
- Prescription cannabinoid medicines have been available since 1985 and have been safely used. However, concerns about tolerability and efficacy have limited the usefulness of these medications.
- Epidiolex (cannabidiol) is a recently approved extraction of CBD from plant sources. Large, well-conducted clinical trials in childhood epilepsies demonstrated an increase in liver enzymes up to three times normal when combined with valproic acid.

Introduction

The clinician should be aware that marijuana and medical marijuana are currently recognized by the US Drug Enforcement Agency (DEA) Comprehensive Drug Abuse Prevention and Control Act of 1970 (Controlled Substances Act) as a Schedule I controlled substance are defined as having a high potential for abuse, no currently accepted medicinal use in treatment in the United States, and a lack of accepted safety data for use of the treatment under medical supervision (Drug Enforcement Administration, 2016).

The US Food and Drug Administration (FDA) has not approved any marketing application for cannabis for the treatment of any disease or condition. However, the cannabis-derived drug product Epidiolex (cannabidiol) has been approved by the FDA in 2018 and, earlier, so have three other synthetic cannabis-related drugs: dronabinol (Marinol and Syndros) and nabilone (Cesamet). Nabiximols (Sativex) is a cannabis-derived drug combination of Δ^9-tetrahydrocannabinol (THC) and cannabidiol (CBD) and recently failed clinical trials in the USA but is available in other countries including Canada and the EU. The FDA has not approved any other cannabis, cannabis-derived or CBD product currently available on the market (US Food and Drug Administration, 2020).

Over 30 million chemicals are listed in the reference textbook *Chemical Abstracts*. However, only around 100 of these compounds are known to have an addictive potential (Gardner, 2014). Despite this small number, addiction remains a serious global public health problem.

People decide how drugs are used and can choose to use them as a remedy for a health concern or to use it as a substance of abuse with potentially severe consequences. Opioids and, to a lesser degree marijuana, are good examples of the need to balance benefits of use with the risk of dependence and addiction. For opioids, this is especially concerning due to the risk of respiratory cessation and death. We are now at the doorstep of a similar challenge with cannabinoids as scientific inquiry and public opinion grapple with the next steps in the journey of development and discovery.

Many consider medical marijuana and cannabis to be a benign drug with few significant risks. However, multiple factors must be considered to fully understand the safety of these molecules and how cannabinoids work. Much of this science, unfortunately, has yet to be studied. The dosage provided, the formulation of the drug and how it is administered, the reason why it is consumed and the expectations of the user, and previous experience are all important factors to determine the safety of a product. For the approved medications, the dosage has been determined by finding the effective dose through controlled clinical trials to treat the targeted medical symptoms. For unapproved cannabis products including medical marijuana, insufficient evidence is available to determine a safe and effective dose. Similarly, for formulation and administration of an approved product, a high level of confidence in the purity and identity of the drug dosed must be present and all cannabinoid-based products are consumed as a spray, capsule or liquid. In contrast, medical marijuana is typically consumed through inhalation through smoking although other routes including oral and transdermal are sometimes used but are inadequately studied. The smoke from inhalation of cannabis is similar to tobacco but usually without nicotine, and includes THC and other cannabinoids, terpenes and flavonoids that are constituents of *Cannabis sativa* (Hoffman et al., 1975). Many of these elements found in smoke are known to be harmful to respiratory tissue and some are carcinogens. Currently, no products smoked by patients for any therapeutic use have been approved.

In Chapter 4 we reviewed the five cannabinoid-based products that have been approved for clinical use starting in 1985. As with all approved pharmaceutical products, the safety and efficacy have been established through high-quality scientific studies and clinical trials and the medicines are monitored for continuing safe use. Although these approved medications are considered safe, the majority of cannabinoid use surprisingly remains with phytocannabinoids and medical marijuana, both of which are unstudied and unapproved by government agencies. Considering the absence of clinical data and the multiple legal hazards associated with cannabis use, it is remarkable that many clinicians remain unfamiliar with the approved products and rarely prescribe them. Likely we will learn more with the recent approval of the CBD product Epidiolex as the safety of this drug is monitored over time by the manufacturer and US and EU regulatory agencies.

For the present, there is considerable safety information already available on marijuana, but the lack of consistency in the mixture of cannabinoids and other constituents including terpenes and flavonoids, which can differ significantly depending on the environment that the plant was cultivated in and the techniques used for harvesting and storage, can significantly affect the end product.

The use of smoked cannabis is clearly associated with respiratory effects including chronic bronchitis, inflammation, emphysema and reduction in pulmonary function. Because of these inherent hazards with smoking, it seems highly unlikely any smoked product will ever be approved for clinical use. There are also other concerns from the existing safety data on marijuana that include cardiovascular effects such as tachycardia, increased blood pressure, cardiomyopathy and myocardial infarction in individuals with preexisting cardiovascular disease. In addition, immunosuppressive effects, sedation (individuals driving under the influence of cannabis are anywhere from two to seven times more likely to be involved in both fatal and nonfatal motor vehicle collisions) and motor coordination effects are all risks associated with cannabis use. Many of these effects are discussed throughout the book and are well reviewed elsewhere but current knowledge has not determined that medical marijuana is safe (Sachs, McGlade and Yurgelun-Todd, 2015).

Other considerations in using medical marijuana include psychological and cognitive effects, drug interactions which have been identified recently in the clinical trials of Epidiolex, and effects of long-term, heavy amounts including tolerance and addiction. Many of these effects will be discussed in the appropriate chapters throughout this book but it is difficult to regard the use of the word "medical" appropriate in the description of marijuana.

Although medical marijuana is not approved, a great deal can be learned from the recent approval of Epidiolex, a CBD product completely extracted from the cannabis plant. During the approval process, results from three high-quality randomized clinical trials have provided considerable information about CBD. Safety concerns were identified in the Epidiolex trials but had to be weighed against the evidence of efficacy in the treatment of children living with a devastating neurological disease in the final approval decision.

As part of any approval process, the US FDA is required to publish in the drug label any safety concerns that arose from the clinical trial data. In the Epidiolex label, the FDA warns about the possibility of hepatocellular injury and elevation of transaminase enzymes from the use of this CBD product. This liver enzyme elevation is especially a concern in the presence of valproate that is used in epilepsy as well as several behavioral and pain conditions. Somnolence and sedation in addition to suicidal behavior and ideation were also listed in the safety warnings. Finally, drug interactions including inhibition of CYP3A4 or CYP2C19 or induction of CYP3A4 or CYP2C19 were listed by the FDA as especially worthy of attention in monitoring patient safety (Greenwich Biosciences, 2018).

We have previously discussed Epidiolex in Chapter 4 and in this chapter we will only have the opportunity to discuss a few other questions regarding the risks of unapproved and unmonitored cannabis. Epidiolex is an excellent example of determining the risk and benefit of a drug and its approval was highly anticipated by the neurological and patient communities. But if we are to use cannabinoids continuing assessment of safety, as with all clinical treatments, will remain necessary.

Despite the gradual legalization of medical marijuana in North America, Europe and Australia and the availability of approved cannabinoid medications, cannabis still remains the most used illicit drug in the world (Anthony, Warner and Kessler, 1997). The United Nations Office of Drugs and Crime (UNODC) in a recent review estimated that over 200 million people annually use cannabis for recreational or medical uses. In the United States, approximately 100 million Americans were estimated to have used cannabis at some time.

With such a large number of users, the question of possible dependency and addiction continues to be an important concern. When contrasted with opioids, nicotine or alcohol, cannabis appears relatively safe for the casual and infrequent user. Approximately 8–10% of these cannabis users will, however, eventually develop drug dependency on cannabis with a lifetime risk estimated at 9%. In comparison, lifetime risk for developing dependency on other drugs is 32% for nicotine, 23% for heroin, 17% for cocaine, 15% for alcohol and 11% for stimulant drugs.

In 2000, Colorado followed the lead of California and legalized medical marijuana and later was the first, in 2012, to allow recreational use of cannabis. To receive permission to receive medical marijuana the individual had to obtain a license for use. In 2008 less than 5000 licenses had been issued for medical marijuana but by 2012 over 100,000 had been approved (Monte, Zane and Heard, 2015; Wang et al., 2018) .

Data from Colorado after legalization of medical and recreational marijuana have shown increased emergency room visits and hospitalizations related to marijuana use. Hall et al. (2018) reported emergency room visits statewide in Colorado between 2012 and 2014 and found a fivefold increase in mental health diagnosis in cannabis-associated visits to the emergency room. Overall, during the same period cannabis-related visits to a group of Colorado hospitals increased almost 40% from 824 per 100,000 to 1146 visits per 100,000 (Hall et al., 2018; Wang et al., 2018).

Although the risk of cannabis dependency today is lower compared with many other drugs, it still remains a major public health issue with potentially devastating consequences for individuals that misuse cannabis or have underlying physical or psychiatric morbidities. In the USA, for example, cannabis use has led to psychiatric hospitalization for dependency or acute intoxication and represents an estimated 16% of hospital admissions. Only abuse of alcohol leads to more admissions for intoxication or dependency (Anthony, Warner and Kessler, 1997). In Europe a similar pattern of use emerges with over 83 million European adults using cannabis and an estimated 11% at risk for dependence (Montanari et al., 2017). As social barriers continue to be lowered and access to high-potency THC made easier, understanding the safety and potential dangers of misuse will become an ever-growing public health need.

The Neurochemistry of Addiction and Cannabinoids

The mesolimbic system within the brain has been identified as the internal reward system and is closely related to the process of addiction. Drugs of abuse including opiates, stimulants, cocaine and alcohol activate this system in the brain. The endocannabinoid system (ECS) shares anatomically many of the pathways of the mesolimbic system and modulates many of the neurotransmitters activated in dependency and addiction.

As we previously reviewed in Chapter 3, endocannabinoids bind to presynaptic cannabinoid receptors and multiple non-cannabinoid receptors critical to intercellular signaling. Glutamate, gamma-aminobutyric acid (GABA) and dopamine are among the neurotransmitters modulated by the ECS and are widely dispersed throughout the mesolimbic system.

The mesolimbic system originates in the ventral tegmental area (VTA), which lies adjacent to the substantia nigra (SN) in the midbrain. Both the VTA and SN are major centers of dopamine in the brain and axons from these neurons stretch along the mesolimbic tract to the basal forebrain and terminate within the nucleus accumbens (NAc). The NAc is generally recognized as part of the internal rewards system but this nucleus also serves other complex functions including processing of aversive stimuli and learning avoidance.

A common feature of drugs of abuse is the release of dopamine in the NAc from activation of the mesolimbic pathway. Within the NAc the inhibitory neurotransmitter GABA is also released and projects back to the dopamine neurons in the midbrain VTA. The NAc also receives input from non-dopamine neurons in the prefrontal cortex, hippocampus and amygdala to release the excitatory neurotransmitter glutamate. The binding of cannabinoid receptor agonists (including endocannabinoids and phytocannabinoids) inhibits the release of the excitatory glutamate into the NAc with subsequent reduction of GABA release in the VTA from neurons originating at higher centers. Through this process, the ECS indirectly disinhibits the release of dopamine in the NAc.

The cannabinoid 1 (CB_1) receptor is highly expressed in these regions that govern the mesolimbic pathways. THC binds to the receptor and activates the VTA–NAc circuit (Diana et al., 1998) increasing dopamine in the NAc similar to other addictive drugs (Di Chiara and Imperato, 1988; Diana et al., 1998). Other studies have added additional support by reporting an increase by THC of dopamine in the NAc in a calcium-dependent manner. This increase of dopamine is blocked by the administration of naloxone (Chen et al., 1990; Tanda, Pontieri and Di Chiara, 1997).

Cannabis Dependence, Tolerance and Withdrawal

In the past, the question of whether cannabis is addictive was a controversial topic. Now there is no disagreement whether dependency, addiction and withdrawal occur with frequent, heavy use of cannabis. Recent editions of DSM-5 and ICD-10 now include criteria to identify these conditions. As clinicians become more familiar with these criteria, an informed perspective will be formed, and the potential risks identified.

Typically, in addiction studies, animal models are employed to assess the addictive potential of a drug. Unfortunately, these models have been difficult to utilize in the evaluation of cannabis for many reasons including the hydrophobic properties of the molecule and difficulty in intravenous administration.

Recent preclinical studies, however, have had better success in overcoming these obstacles and have confirmed the addictive properties of cannabis. Two frequently employed preclinical models that are used to assess dependency risks include the conditioned place preference (CPP) test and the self-administration of drug. The CPP is an animal model that determines the strength of environmental cues to produce drug-seeking behavior and results from animal studies have demonstrated qualitative outcomes for cannabis similar to the opiates and other drugs of addiction (Gardner, 2014). Self-administration is evaluated by training animals on a predetermined fixed frequency for intravenous drug administration. Animals then learn to titrate the dose of the addictive drug to maintain the desired level (Justinova et al., 2004).

Increasing dosage or potency of a drug typically increases the addictive potential of the molecule. The increased potency of cannabis over the past few decades have led many to speculate that these trends contribute to the increase in diagnosis of cannabis use disorder (Piomelli et al., 2018). Once controversial, human studies clearly have demonstrated the dependency and addictive qualities of cannabis. Previous research comparing preference in subjects allowed to choose between active marijuana and placebo marijuana have confirmed research participants preference for active drug and increased dosage also increases the preference for drug (Chait and Zacny, 1992; Haney et al., 1997, 1999). The development of dependence on cannabis is now a well-established scientific fact for patients exposed to high concentrations of THC over an extended use.

Withdrawal effects from the abrupt sensation of cannabis have also been reported in several studies. In one early study, THC was provided orally to users who smoked cannabis. After two weeks, the THC was abruptly terminated and within 6 hours the subjects complained of "inner unrest." After 12 hours the subjects also reported discomfort including increased irritability, insomnia and restlessness. Symptoms were also observed including sweating, rhinorrhea, loose stools, hiccups and anorexia. Higher doses of THC before stopping administration resulted in greater symptoms of withdrawal. When cannabis use was resumed in these subjects, symptoms abated (Jones, Benowitz and Bachman, 1976). A similar study followed several years later using high-dose smoked cannabis for four weeks. With abrupt termination of the smoked cannabis, similar withdrawal symptoms were reported in the first week of washout (Georgotas and Zeidenberg, 1979).

Clinical Aspects of Abuse and Withdrawal

Subsequent work has reaffirmed the presence of withdrawal that varies in severity and duration based upon usage of the cannabis. Irritability, craving, sleep disturbance and appetite reduction occurs within 24 hours of termination of cannabis and may persist for several weeks (Haney, 2005). In randomized double-blind studies of readministration of cannabis or THC, symptoms were consistently relieved (Haney et al., 1999; Stephens, Roffman and Curtin, 2000).

To date, no medications have been approved for the treatment of cannabis withdrawal. Several studies using currently approved cannabinoid-agonist medications have been completed. Nabilone, previously discussed in Chapter 4, is a synthetic analog of THC and was first studied in 2013 for withdrawal in cannabis smokers. Doses of 6–8 mg/d were provided with observed reduction in complaints of irritability. Sleep and appetite were both reported to improve with minor psychomotor side effects noted at the higher dose. Importantly, although nabilone is a CB_1 agonist, experienced subjects did not report "liking" the drug (Cooper et al., 2013). A follow-up study of subjects provided smoked cannabis compared placebo, zolpidem 12.5 mg HS and a combination of zolpidem 12.5 mg HS plus nabilone at

3 mg PO BID upon cessation of cannabis. Both medication conditions decreased withdrawal-related disruptions in sleep, but only zolpidem in combination with nabilone decreased withdrawal-related disruptions in mood and food intake relative to placebo. Zolpidem in combination with nabilone also decreased self-administration of active cannabis, but zolpidem alone did not. Zolpidem in combination with nabilone also produced small increases in certain abuse-related subjective capsule ratings, while zolpidem alone did not. Neither medication condition showed changes in cognition (Haney *et al.*, 2013).

Dronabinol, a synthetic THC, has also been evaluated as a possible treatment for cannabis withdrawal. In one well-controlled, double-blind, placebo-controlled 12-week study 156 cannabis-dependent adults were randomized to either 20 mg of dronabinol BID or placebo. Although there was no difference in abstinence rates after the end of the maintenance phase, withdrawal symptoms were considerably lower on dronabinol (Levin *et al.*, 2011).

Nabiximols has also been studied as an agonist treatment for cannabis withdrawal. Unlike nabilone and dronabinol, nabiximols is a combination of extracts of THC and CBD from the cannabis plant. In a six- to eight-week, randomized, double-blind clinical trial on treatment of cannabis withdrawal, nabiximols attenuated symptoms and was superior to placebo in reducing the overall severity. However, reduced cannabis use for both drug and placebo groups was reported at follow-up (Allsop *et al.*, 2014).

In another study of fixed and self-titration of nabiximols compared with placebo, the drug was found to significantly reduce cannabis withdrawal symptoms with the exception of the symptom of craving. However, both placebo and nabiximols showed no difference in the reduction of craving (Trigo *et al.*, 2016).

There has been a continuing interest in the potential usefulness of CBD alone in cannabis withdrawal. The actions of CBD often reduce or counteract the effects of THC and in one study that provided CBD to subjects using smoked THC, the psychotropic effects were reported to be reduced (Dalton *et al.*, 1976). Similar results were found in reducing complaints of oral THC intoxication with the addition of oral CBD (Zuardi *et al.*, 1982).

A more recent study reassessed the effects of oral CBD on smoked cannabis. In a multisite, double-blind, placebo-controlled study, 31 cannabis smokers were treated with placebo or CBD doses of 200 mg, 400 mg or 800 mg capsules. No effects of CBD compared with placebo in the subjective, reinforcing or cardiovascular effects of the smoked cannabis were reported (Haney *et al.*, 2016).

Tolerance develops when the effect of the drug diminishes, and higher doses are required for the original effect. Earlier studies during the 1970s on smoked and oral cannabis demonstrated tolerance with repeated exposure to the drug. In one study cannabis users were given 21 mg oral THC for 30 days and were compared with healthy controls. Signs of intoxication and elevation in mood declined along with cognitive and cardiovascular function over the course of the study (Jones, Benowitz and Bachman, 1976). When subjects on oral THC completed the study, the cannabinoid was abruptly withdrawn. After 6 hours "inner unrest" was reported and within 12 hours subjects were observed with increased activity and restlessness, irritability and insomnia. A second study followed a few years later and affirmed that the elevated self-ratings disappeared after several days with smoked cannabis. When the smoked cannabis was discontinued, a withdrawal consistent with earlier studies was observed (Georgotas and Zeidenberg, 1979).

Other studies, however, in animals and humans have reported mixed results when stopping cannabis after chronic use (Wikler, 1976; Compton, Dewey and Martin, 1990).

The addition of THC to reduce withdrawal effects from cannabis has similarly met with inconsistent findings.

Several changes in the CB_1 receptor likely underlie the development of tolerance. Desensitization of the receptor occurs when binding to the CB_1 receptor is disconnected from the intracellular processes and receptor downregulation also occurs where the receptor is internalized into the cell and broken down. Both processes are in evidence with tolerance to cannabinoids. The development of tolerance is further complicated with the development of regional variation in different regions of the brain and body (McKinney *et al.*, 2008). Since cannabinoids have multiple effects, this regional variation can unfold across unrelated therapeutic areas. Perception, cognition, anxiety, mood, interocular pressure (IOP), electroencephalogram (EEG) and psychomotor effects have all been found to be altered as tolerance and withdrawal unfold (Compton, Dewey and Martin, 1990; Gorelick *et al.*, 2013). One example would be cardiovascular tolerance and withdrawal through heart rate and blood pressure that can demonstrate significant variation. Tolerance to the sedating effects of cannabis is another effect reported with significant variability (Schierenbeck *et al.*, 2008) although the data are very limited.

Although it is now clear that persistent cannabis use can result in tolerance and withdrawal, this has not been observed with the approved cannabinoid products. There are several reasons that could account for this finding including nabilone and dronabinol are generally approved for acute medical complaints such as chemotherapy-induced nausea and vomiting (CINV) where the dosage is both limited and low. In instances in long-term treatment such as anorexia related to HIV, dependence and tolerance is rarely reported.

Further, tolerance has also not been reported in other areas such as chronic pain associated with spasticity. Nabiximols, approved in some countries for the treatment of pain associated with spasticity, has not been found to develop tolerance. One open-label extension study after a five-week trial of nabiximols in multiple sclerosis patients in central pain, found no significant difference in the extended use of the analgesic benefit. In another open-label, long-term study of multiple sclerosis with spasticity, a similar replication of analgesic effect was found (Serpell, Notcutt and Collin, 2013).

Cannabinoids and Neurodevelopment

Cannabinoids are known to have complex effects on the maturing nervous system with both neurotoxic and neuroprotective properties identified at different times of development in various tissue within the central nervous system. Exposure to phytocannabinoids and endocannabinoids is known to disrupt the development of the immature nervous system and result in harmful outcomes (Arseneault *et al.*, 2004).

Although the human data remains limited in understanding these effects, animal studies have provided important insights on how cannabinoids are harmful to normal neurodevelopment. It is now well established that CB_1 receptor activation during development results in disruption of neural cell communication and survival (Downer and Campbell, 2010; Chiarlone *et al.*, 2014). When THC is administered to cell cultures of neural tissue, cell damage (including shrinkage of cell bodies and disruption of DNA) and death have been observed. THC has been found to be especially toxic at high doses to cell cultures of hippocampus while cortical neurons are affected at both high and low doses (Campbell, 2001). In contrast, CBD has been found to be neuroprotective in developing neurons in hippocampus and cortex and in the adult rodent cerebrum (Hampson *et al.*, 1998; Hayakawa *et al.*, 2007).

Chronic administration of cannabinoids in laboratory animals has found dose-dependent neuronal damage in multiple locations with high expressions of the CB_1 receptor including the hippocampus and other limbic structures. Examples of damage to developing neural tissue include reduction in chemical synapses, shrinkage of cell bodies and reduction in cell density and length. In humans, these disruptions may result in unwanted cognitive and emotional results demonstrated later in adolescence and adulthood (Jutras-Aswad *et al.*, 2009).

Several neuroimaging studies and a postmortem examination have been performed in humans with chronic cannabis use. Imaging studies are mixed demonstrating little to no effect in some reports and significant differences in brain volume in others. Generally, patients with longer exposure to cannabinoids at higher doses demonstrate changes similar to the animal studies. Reductions in hippocampal and amygdala volume and cerebellar white matter have been reported (Yücel *et al.*, 2008; Solowij *et al.*, 2011).

In a postmortem study, CB_1 receptor expression and integrity was disrupted in chronic cannabinoid users (Villares, 2007). The hippocampus, basal ganglia and mesencephalon of chronic users were found to be the most damaged areas with reduction of mRNA.

Cannabinoids and Psychosis

There is little disagreement that psychosis can occur while using cannabinoids. Recognized for thousands of years for its ability to induce paranoia and delusions, the French psychiatrist J. J. Moreau brought this phenomenon into modern medicine in 1845 with the recognition of the psychoactive properties of hashish.

Usually the psychosis is mild and limited to a short period of intoxication. However, whether THC can precipitate chronic psychotic symptoms in individuals or increase the incidence or severity of psychiatric illness remains an important question.

In a three-day, double-blind, randomized study, 22 healthy subjects with a prior history of cannabis use but never diagnosed with cannabis use disorder were given placebo, 2.5 mg THC or 5.0 mg THC through an intravenous line. Behavioral, cognitive and endocrine effects were measured during the study and follow-up interviews were conducted at one, three and six months. Intravenous administration over 2 minutes was chosen to minimize the inter- and intravariability of inhaled THC. Positive symptoms including hallucinations, delusions, disorganized activity and a formal thought disorder quickly followed and persisted for up to 1 hour. The negative symptoms of affective flattening and apathy were also induced and followed a similar time course. Unlike other drug-induced (e.g. amphetamine, dopamine agonists, serotonergic agents, LSD) psychotic episodes that produce only positive symptoms, THC more closely produced the broader spectrum of symptoms seen in schizophrenia including negative and cognitive symptoms. Subjects followed up over six months did not report any persistent complaints (D'Souza *et al.*, 2004).

A more important (and controversial) question is whether exposure to cannabis can increase the risk of future psychotic symptoms and schizophrenia. Studies of individual patients have not been useful in this question as it is difficult to predict the likelihood of symptoms and occurrence in any one person. Population studies, however, have provided important information on the risk of developing schizophrenia associated with cannabis use.

Using the Swedish national health database, investigators were able to screen 50,000 conscripts into the Swedish military in 1969 and follow them for 15 years. All draftees were interviewed during entry into the military by a psychiatrist or psychologist to identify any psychiatric disorders and inquire about any cannabis use. A dose–response association was noted between cannabis use at conscription and subsequent diagnosis of schizophrenia. Only 362 subjects were admitted to a psychiatric hospital for schizophrenia and only 18 of these individuals used cannabis alone (Andréasson et al., 1987; Zammit et al., 2002).

Other population-based studies were to follow from New Zealand (Arseneault et al., 2004), the Netherlands (van Os et al., 2002) and elsewhere providing evidence that cannabis use increases the risk of developing a psychotic disorder (Zammit et al., 2008). In the last few years observational studies and several meta-analyses have been published that further provide information on the risk of developing a psychotic disorder. In one observational study in the UK, it was reported that the effects of cannabis differed based upon the habits of the individual. High-frequency, high-potency cannabis users had a greatest risk for relapse and more severe symptoms compared with those that used a less potent cannabis less frequently. In a recent meta-analysis, 35 studies were reviewed and found a consistent dose–response effect with greater risk for a psychotic illness with those that used cannabis frequently. From these studies, individuals have a 40% increase risk to develop a psychotic disorder if they ever used cannabis. For those using more frequent cannabis, the increased risk was estimated to be between 50% and 200% (Moore et al., 2007). Earlier cannabis use in early adolescence (before age 15) seems to place the individual at greater risk for developing a psychotic disorder and those using higher potency to become symptomatic earlier (Large et al., 2011).

Concluding Thoughts

Cannabis is the most commonly used illicit drug in the United States and it is estimated 7.5% of the US population aged greater than 12 years of age reported using cannabis one month before the survey (National Institute on Drug Abuse, 2019). The prevalence of marijuana use increased among persons aged 18 years or older but use among those between 12 and 17 years has not changed. Although it is difficult to know how much of this use is driven by the desire to use marijuana for a valid medical purpose or for recreation, one survey reported use of marijuana in adults with medical conditions to be greater than that in those without (Lankenau et al., 2018). In the survey 11.2% of young adults with medical conditions reported using marijuana on a daily basis to relieve the symptoms of asthma, chronic obstructive pulmonary disease, arthritis, cancer and depression.

With the approval of prescription cannabinoid-based medications available for over 30 years, an obvious question is the relationship between the medications reviewed in this chapter and medical marijuana. Approved products are placed into schedules to regulate the risk and benefit of the drug. In the United States, for example, the synthetic THC Marinol is assigned Schedule III, Syndros Schedule II and THC extracted from the cannabis plant Schedule I. In all instances the THC molecule is identical. Despite these legal restrictions on THC, in the United States as of mid-2019, medical marijuana has been legalized in 33 states and the District of Columbia. Globally over 30 countries including Canada, the UK and Germany allow marijuana to be used for medical purposes. There has been a great deal of experience with medical marijuana but the lack of controls in ingredients, concentration, means of delivery, coadministration with other substances and no long-term data makes comparison with approved medications impossible to complete.

Despite this uncertainty, many patients prefer medical marijuana over available prescription cannabinoids. This is noteworthy considering prescription cannabinoids may potentially be reimbursed under insurance plans and significant legal restrictions and social approbation may exist with non-prescription marijuana.

In May 2019 the FDA held a public hearing to hear presentations on the use of cannabis or cannabis-derived products (US Food and Drug Administration, 2019). Testimony presented reported in a large consumer survey that one in every four adults in the USA had tried CBD once within the last 24 months. One in seven responders reported the use of daily CBD for a variety of complaints including stress, anxiety and joint pain. Respondents felt that CBD was effective and safe. Half the respondents reported that CBD was very effective for sleep.

The FDA has recognized the growing availability and use of CBD although any product extracted from cannabis still is Schedule I. This was made more confusing with the passage in 2018 by Congress of legislation referred to as the "Farm Bill." In this law Congress removed hemp, defined as cannabis and cannabis derivatives with low concentrations of THC (less than 0.03% dry weight cannabis), from Schedule I. Thus, when CBD is extracted from the cannabis plant containing THC above this concentration, it is regarded as a Schedule I drug and enforced as a drug with any high abuse potential. The Schedule I drugs include heroin, LSD, MDMA (ecstasy), among others. In contrast, if the same molecule of CBD is separated from hemp (with concentration of THC less than or equal to 0.03%), it is considered safe and unscheduled by the FDA.

As noted previously in this chapter, the FDA has approved CBD marketed as Epidiolex for the treatment of rare severe childhood epilepsies. Epidiolex had to demonstrate purity and stability in addition to efficacy to obtain approval and its place in Schedule V by the FDA. No other CBD products have been approved by the FDA and several warning letters have been issued to manufacturers of these unapproved products to stop their commercial activities.

Additional testimony addressed concerns regarding contaminates and potential health hazards in CBD products not approved by the FDA. One speaker noted that there was + or − 20% variation in the CBD amount published on the label of products. Another presenter noted an even broader variation from 0% to 70% content of CBD that was listed on the label. Testing for lead in CBD products was reported in another presentation as 34 parts per billion. In comparison, the US Environmental Protection Agency (EPA) published guidelines in 1991 for lead contamination in water of 15 parts per billion (US Food and Drug Administration, 2019).

Bibliography

Allsop, D. J. et al. (2014) 'Nabiximols as an agonist replacement therapy during cannabis withdrawal: a randomized clinical trial', JAMA Psychiatry, 71(3), 281–291. doi:10.1001/jamapsychiatry.2013.3947.

Andréasson, S. et al. (1987) 'Cannabis and schizophrenia. A longitudinal study of Swedish conscripts', The Lancet, 330(8574), 1483–1486. doi:10.1016/S0140-6736(87) 92620-1.

Anthony, J. C., Warner, L. A. and Kessler, R. C. (1997) 'Comparative epidemiology of dependence on tobacco, alcohol, controlled substances, and inhalants: basic findings from the National Comorbidity Survey.', in G. A. Marlatt and G. R. VandenBos (eds.), Addictive Behaviors: Readings on Etiology, Prevention, and Treatment. Washington:

American Psychological Association, pp. 3–39. doi:10.1037/10248-001.

Arseneault, L. et al. (2004) 'Causal association between cannabis and psychosis: examination of the evidence', British Journal of Psychiatry, 184(2), 110–117. doi:10.1192/bjp.184.2.110.

Campbell, V. A. (2001) 'Tetrahydrocannabinol-induced apoptosis of cultured cortical neurones is associated with cytochrome c release and caspase-3 activation', Neuropharmacology, 40(5), 702–709. doi:10.1016/S0028-3908(00)00210-0.

Chait, L. D. and Zacny, J. P. (1992) 'Reinforcing and subjective effects of oral Δ9-THC and smoked marijuana in humans', Psychopharmacology, 107(2–3), 255–262. doi:10.1007/BF02245145.

Chen, J. et al. (1990) 'Δ9-Tetrahydrocannabinol produces naloxone-blockable enhancement of presynaptic basal dopamine efflux in nucleus accumbens of conscious, freely-moving rats as measured by intracerebral microdialysis', Psychopharmacology, 102(2), 156–162. doi:10.1007/BF02245916.

Chiarlone, A. et al. (2014) 'A restricted population of CB_1 cannabinoid receptors with neuroprotective activity', Proceedings of the National Academy of Sciences of the United States of America, 111(22), 8257–8262. doi:10.1073/pnas.1400988111.

Compton, D. R., Dewey, W. L. and Martin, B. R. (1990) 'Cannabis dependence and tolerance production', Advances in Alcohol and Substance Abuse, 9(1–2), 129–147. doi:10.1080/J251v09n01_08.

Cooper, Z. D. et al. (2013) 'A human laboratory study investigating the effects of quetiapine on marijuana withdrawal and relapse in daily marijuana smokers', Addiction Biology, 18(6), 993–1002. doi:10.1111/j.1369-1600.2012.00461.x.

Dalton, W. S. et al. (1976) 'Influence of cannabidiol on delta-9-tetrahydrocannabinol effects', Clinical Pharmacology & Therapeutics, 19(3), 300–309. doi:10.1002/cpt1976193300.

Di Chiara, G. and Imperato, A. (1988) 'Drugs abused by humans preferentially increase synaptic dopamine concentrations in the mesolimbic system of freely moving rats', Proceedings of the National Academy of Sciences of the United States of America, 85 (14), 5274–5278. doi:10.1073/pnas.85.14.5274.

Diana, M. et al. (1998) 'Mesolimbic dopaminergic decline after cannabinoid withdrawal', Proceedings of the National Academy of Sciences of the United States of America, 95(17), 10269–10273. doi:10.1073/pnas.95.17.10269.

Downer, E. J. and Campbell, V. A. (2010) 'Phytocannabinoids, CNS cells and development: a dead issue?', Drug and Alcohol Review, 29(1), 91–98. doi:10.1111/j.1465-3362.2009.00102.x.

Drug Enforcement Administration (2016). Title 21 United States Code (USC) Controlled Substances Act. Available at: www.deadiversion.usdoj.gov/21cfr/21usc/812.htm (Accessed: May 26, 2020).

D'Souza, D.C. et al. (2004) 'The psychotomimetic effects of intravenous delta-9-tetrahydrocannabinol in healthy individuals: implications for psychosis', Neuropsychopharmacology, 29, 1558–1572. doi:10.1038/sj.npp.1300496.

Gardner, E. (2014) 'Cannabinoids and addiction', in R. Pertwee, (ed)., Handbook of Cannabis. Oxford: Oxford University Press, pp. 173–188.

Georgotas, A. and Zeidenberg, P. (1979) 'Observations on the effects of four weeks of heavy marihuana smoking on group interaction and individual behavior', Comprehensive Psychiatry, 20(5), 427–432. doi:10.1016/0010-440X(79)90027-0.

Gorelick, D. A. et al. (2013) 'Tolerance to effects of high-dose oral Δ9-tetrahydrocannabinol and plasma cannabinoid concentrations in male daily cannabis smokers', Journal of Analytical Toxicology, 37(1), 11–16. doi:10.1093/jat/bks081.

Greenwich Biosciences (2018) Epidiolex® (cannabidiol). Carlsbad, CA: Greenwich Biosciences, Inc. Available at: www.epidiolexhcp.com/themes/custom/epidiolex_hcp/files/factsheet.pdf (Accessed: May 30, 2020).

Hall, K. E. et al. (2018) 'Mental health-related emergency department visits associated with cannabis in Colorado', Academic Emergency

Medicine, 25(5), 526–537. doi:10.1111/acem.13393.

Hampson, A. J. *et al.* (1998) 'Cannabidiol and (−)Δ⁹-tetrahydrocannabinol are neuroprotective antioxidants', *Proceedings of the National Academy of Sciences of the United States of America*, 95(14), 8268–8273. https://doi.org/10.1073/pnas.95.14.8268.

Haney, M. (2005) 'The marijuana withdrawal syndrome: diagnosis and treatment', *Current Psychiatry Reports*, 7(5), 360–366. doi:10.1007/s11920-005-0036-1.

Haney, M. *et al.* (1997) 'Factors influencing marijuana self-administration by humans', *Behavioural Pharmacology*, 8(2–3), 101–112.

Haney, M. *et al.* (1999) 'Abstinence symptoms following oral THC administration to humans', *Psychopharmacology*, 141(4), 385–394. doi:10.1007/s002130050848.

Haney, M. *et al.* (2013) 'Nabilone decreases marijuana withdrawal and a laboratory measure of marijuana relapse', *Neuropsychopharmacology*, 38(8), 1557–1565. doi:10.1038/npp.2013.54.

Haney, M. *et al.* (2016) 'Oral cannabidiol does not alter the subjective, reinforcing or cardiovascular effects of smoked cannabis', *Neuropsychopharmacology*, 41(8), 1974–1982. doi:10.1038/npp.2015.367.

Hayakawa, K. *et al.* (2007) 'Repeated treatment with cannabidiol but not Δ9-tetrahydrocannabinol has a neuroprotective effect without the development of tolerance', *Neuropharmacology*, 52(4), 1079–1087. doi:10.1016/j.neuropharm.2006.11.005.

Hoffman, D. *et al.* (1975) 'On the carcinogenicity of marijuana smoke', in V. C. Runekles (ed.), *Recent Advances in Phytochemistry*. New York: Plenum Press. pp. 63–81.

Jones, R. T., Benowitz, N. and Bachman, J. (1976) 'Clinical studies of cannabis tolerance and dependence', *Annals of the New York Academy of Sciences*, 282(1), 221–239. doi:10.1111/j.1749-6632.1976.tb49901.x.

Justinova, Z. *et al.* (2004) 'The opioid antagonist naltrexone reduces the reinforcing effects of Δ⁹-tetrahydrocannabinol (THC) in squirrel monkeys', *Psychopharmacology*, 173(1), 186–194. doi:10.1007/s00213-003-1693-6.

Jutras-Aswad, D. *et al.* (2009) 'Neurobiological consequences of maternal cannabis on human fetal development and its neuropsychiatric outcome', *European Archives of Psychiatry and Clinical Neuroscience*, 259(7), 395–412. doi:10.1007/s00406-009-0027-z.

Lankenau, S. E. *et al.* (2018) 'Health conditions and motivations for marijuana use among adult medical marijuana patients and non-patient marijuana users', *Drug and Alcohol Review*, 37(2), 237–246. doi:10.1111/dar.12534.

Large, M. *et al.* (2011) 'Cannabis use and earlier onset of psychosis: a systematic meta-analysis', *Archives of General Psychiatry*, 68(6), 555–561.

Levin, F. R. *et al.* (2011) 'Dronabinol for the treatment of cannabis dependence: a randomized, double-blind, placebo-controlled trial', *Drug and Alcohol Dependence*, 116(1–3), 142–150. doi:10.1016/drugalcdep.2010.12.010.

McKinney, D. L. *et al.* (2008) 'Dose-related differences in the regional pattern of cannabinoid receptor adaptation and in vivo tolerance development to Δ⁹-tetrahydrocannabinol', *Journal of Pharmacology and Experimental Therapeutics*, 324(2), 664–673. doi:10.1124/jpet.107.130328.

Montanari, L. *et al.* (2017) 'Cannabis use among people entering drug treatment in Europe: a growing phenomenon?', *European Addiction Research*, 23(3), 113–121. doi:10.1159/000475810.

Monte, A. A., Zane, R. D. and Heard, K. J. (2015) 'The implications of marijuana legalization in Colorado', *JAMA: Journal of the American Medical Association*, 313(3), 241–242. doi:10.1001/jama.2014.17057.

Moore, T. H. *et al.* (2007) 'Cannabis use and risk of psychotic or affective mental health outcomes: a systematic review', *Lancet*, 370(9584), 319–328. doi:10.1016/S0140-6736(07)61162-3.

National Institute on Drug Abuse (2019) *Monitoring the Future Survey: High School and Youth Trends*, Revised December 2019. Available at www.drugabuse.gov/publications/drugfacts/monitoring-future-survey-high-school-youth-trends (Accessed: June 8, 2020).

Piomelli, D. *et al.* (2018) 'Cannabis and the opioid crisis', *Cannabis and Cannabinoid Research*, 3(1), 108–116. doi:10.1089/can.2018.29011.rtl.

Sachs, J., McGlade, E. and Yurgelun-Todd, D. (2015) 'Safety and toxicology of cannabinoids', *Neurotherapeutics*, 12(4), 735–746. doi:10.1007/s13311-015-0380-8.

Schierenbeck, T. *et al.* (2008) 'Effect of illicit recreational drugs upon sleep: cocaine, ecstasy and marijuana', *Sleep Medicine Reviews*, 12(5), 381–389. doi:10.1016/j.smrv.2007.12.004.

Serpell, M. G., Notcutt, W. and Collin, C. (2013) 'Sativex long-term use: an open-label trial in patients with spasticity due to multiple sclerosis', *Journal of Neurology*, 260(1), 285–295. doi:10.1007/s00415-012-6634-z.

Solowij, N. *et al.* (2011) 'Does cannabis cause lasting brain damage?' in D. Castle, R. M. Murray and D. C. D'Souza (eds.), *Marijuana and Madness*, 2nd ed. Cambridge: Cambridge University Press, pp. 103–113. doi:10.1017/CBO9780511706080.010.

Stephens, R. S., Roffman, R. A. and Curtin, L. (2000) 'Comparison of extended versus brief treatments for marijuana use', *Journal of Consulting and Clinical Psychology*, 68(5), 898–908. doi:10.1037/0022-006X.68.5.898.

Tanda, G., Pontieri, F. E. and Di Chiara, G. (1997) 'Cannabinoid and heroin activation of mesolimbic dopamine transmission by a common μ_1 opioid receptor mechanism', *Science*, 276(5321), 2048–2050. doi:10.1126/science.276.5321.2048.

Trigo, J. M. *et al.* (2016) 'Effects of fixed or self-titrated dosages of Sativex on cannabis withdrawal and cravings', *Drug and Alcohol Dependence*, 161, 298–306. doi:10.1016/j.drugalcdep.2016.02.020.

US Food and Drug Administration (2019). 'Scientific Data and Information about Products Containing Cannabis or Cannabis-Derived Compounds; Public Hearing May 31, 2019'. Available at: www.fda.gov/news-events/fda-meetings-conferences-and-workshops/scientific-data-and-information-about-products-containing-cannabis-or-cannabis-derived-compounds (Accessed: May 27, 2020).

US Food and Drug Administration (2020). *FDA and Cannabis: Research and Drug Approval Process*. Available at: www.fda.gov/news-events/public-health-focus/fda-and-cannabis-research-and-drug-approval-process (Accessed: May 26, 2020).

van Os, J. *et al.* (2002) 'Cannabis use and psychosis: a longitudinal population-based study', *American Journal of Epidemiology*, 156(4), 319–327. doi:10.1093/aje/kwf043.

Villares, J. (2007) 'Chronic use of marijuana decreases cannabinoid receptor binding and mRNA expression in the human brain', *Neuroscience*, 145(1), 323–334. doi:10.1016/j.neuroscience.2006.11.012.

Wang, G. S. *et al.* (2018) 'Marijuana and acute health care contacts in Colorado', *Preventive Medicine*, 104, 24–30. doi:10.1016/j.ypmed.2017.03.022.Marijuana.

Wikler, A. (1976) 'Aspects of tolerance to and dependence on cannabis', *Annals of the New York Academy of Sciences*, 282(1), 126–147. doi:10.1111/j.1749-6632.1976.tb49893.x.

Yücel, M. *et al.* (2008) 'Regional brain abnormalities associated with long-term heavy cannabis use', *Archives of General Psychiatry*, 65(6), 694–701. doi:10.1001/archpsyc.65.6.694.

Zammit, S. *et al.* (2002) 'Self reported cannabis use as a risk factor for schizophrenia in Swedish conscripts of 1969: historical cohort study', *British Medical Journal*, 325(7374), 1199–1201. doi:10.1136/bmj.325.7374.1199.

Zammit, S. *et al.* (2008) 'Effects of cannabis use on outcomes of psychotic disorders: systematic review', *British Journal of Psychiatry*, 193(5), 357–363. doi:10.1192/bjp.bp.107.046375.

Zuardi, A. W. *et al.* (1982) 'Action of cannabidiol on the anxiety and other effects produced by Δ9-THC in normal subjects', *Psychopharmacology*, 76(3), 245–250.

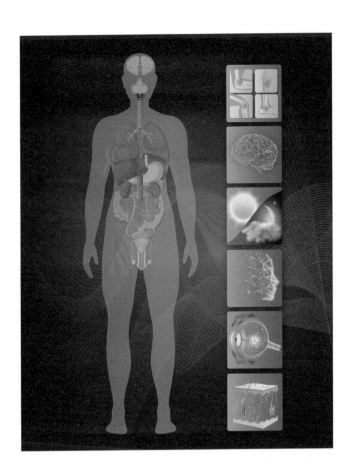

Chapter

6

Cannabinoids and Pain

Pain is as diverse as man. One suffers as one can.
Victor Hugo, Les Miserables

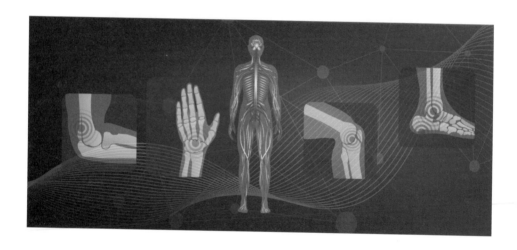

- Pain is the most common complaint of patients that use medical marijuana. Clinical trials of phytocannabinoids and prescription cannabinoids have been generally supportive of their usefulness as an analgesic in chronic pain.
- Treatment with several cannabinoids including Δ^9-tetrahydrocannabinol (THC) and nabilone has not been shown to be effective in postoperative acute pain.
- Cannabinoids and opioids have shared actions in pain relief. Results demonstrating opioid sparing in the presence of cannabinoids are promising but limited to small trial size. Both cannabinoid (CB_1 and CB_2) receptors may moderate this effect.
- Early reports of reduced opioid overdose deaths when using medical marijuana have not been sustained in later epidemiology studies.
- Cannabidiol (CBD) has been demonstrated to be effective in animal models of chronic pain.
- Animal models strongly support cannabinoid effects in experimentally induced acute pain studies but results are mixed in human studies of experimentally induced acute pain treated with nabilone, smoked cannabis or oral THC.

Introduction

In this chapter we will review selected preclinical and clinical studies that may lead to future development of cannabinoids as treatment for pain conditions. Although there are other therapeutic areas where cannabinoids potentially might one day be used, currently the only approvals of cannabinoid-based products have been medications that influence the central nervous system (CNS). Earlier we reviewed in Chapter 4 approvals for cannabinoid-based medicines from the US Food and Drug Administration (FDA), Canada Health and the European Medicines Agency (EMA) as well as other countries for indications that include pain. Nabiximols is used in more countries for pain than any other cannabinoid-based drug although in the USA it recently failed clinical trials for use in relieving cancer pain and is not available for any use.

As approved medications, cannabinoid-based medicines are available by prescription for patient use today. However, as a group, they have not been widely used as concerns regarding efficacy and tolerability have limited their acceptance. However, promise remains for other therapeutic uses in the CNS including neurodegenerative diseases such as Parkinson's disease and amyotrophic lateral sclerosis (ALS), Alzheimer's disease, stroke, schizophrenia, depression and anxiety. Our knowledge is incomplete, and much remains to be accomplished.

Medical marijuana is now available in many countries even though there is absence of both high-quality randomized clinical trials (RCTs) and approval by any regulatory agency worldwide. Despite this gap in knowledge, there is a pressing medical need to treat neuropsychiatric disease and medical marijuana is heavily promoted as treatments for these inadequately treated conditions. For the clinician, weighing the potential benefits of using the available cannabinoids against the potential safety concerns is a frequent challenge. The emerging science is intriguing and promising and deserves further study. However, the safety of the patient should always be prioritized before making any recommendation for treatment where information is incomplete, including the cannabinoids.

Cannabis has long been associated in history as a remedy for pain. Ancient Chinese and Indian reports describe the use of cannabis for rheumatic and gynecological disorders and surgical anesthesia was provided by a mixture of hemp resin and wine. Other stories of the analgesic qualities of cannabis can be found in a publication in 1890 by Russell Reynolds, personal physician of Queen Victoria, for the treatment of menstrual cramps, although the paper was published when the queen was 60 years old and she was likely not the subject of the report (Reynolds, 1890).

Although historical records sometimes are anecdotal with limited information, there is no controversy that cannabis today is a popular treatment for pain. In a recent survey of state registries of medical cannabis in the USA, 67.5% of patients reported chronic pain as the primary complaint. Of this group, 85.5% had substantial or conclusive evidence of improvement. Multiple sclerosis (MS), nausea, cancer and post-traumatic stress disorder, conditions often presenting with pain, were other conditions less frequently associated with medical cannabis use (Boehnke et al., 2019).

Acute pain is a transient insult to the body that involves the stimulation of the peripheral nervous system lasting for an arbitrary period such as up to three months to six months. Chronic pain, in contrast, may persist for an indefinite duration and is generally classified as nociceptive or neuropathic. Nociceptive pain, from the Latin "nocere" meaning "to harm or to hurt," is the perception by specialized nerve endings (nociceptors) of noxious stimuli that potentially may damage the body. Neuropathic pain is damage directly to the neurons in the nociceptive pathways and is often the result of underlying diseases including diabetes, HIV, infection (shingles, postherpetic) or damage from treatments including chemotherapy-induced neuropathy (Nestler, Hyman and Malenka, 2001). Although pain is a complex sensory and behavioral response to irritating stimuli, chronic pain persists independently of the injury and frequently presents a serious clinical challenge to treat.

Cannabinoids (both phytocannabinoids and endocannabinoids) play critical roles in pain and animal studies have demonstrated that cannabinoids can effectively relieve pain in acute and chronic models. High-quality RCTs are demanding and difficult to design in any therapeutic area and are especially challenging in pain. Reliance on highly subjective measures including pain intensity and relief, high placebo effects and poor recruitment may lead to study failures or misleading results. With cannabinoids the added variability between plant-based and synthetic source, dosage, and consistency in delivery as a smoked product, oromucosal spray, oral or ingested formulation make interpretation of results and comparisons sometimes impossible. Finally, the regulatory and legal barriers to obtain and study cannabinoids further delay and discourage research in this area (Finniss et al., 2010).

As a result, human studies utilizing a variety of approaches including uncontrolled and unblinded studies, experimentally induced pain, RCTs and observational research have been mixed in their findings. Despite evidence from preclinical studies showing promising results in acute and chronic pain models, in human trials effectiveness of cannabinoids has been shown in several small chronic pain studies but not in acute pain.

Despite these many challenges to assess the effect of cannabinoids in pain, several reviews of RCTs and meta-analyses have been published. Meta-analyses can be useful in organizing multiple studies in pain with differences in study design and indication to understand the effect of cannabinoids in pain conditions. Since 2000, multiple reviews have been conducted and five meta-analyses are available (Aviram and Samuelly-Leichtag, 2017). One recent meta-analysis by Whiting et al. (2015) used the highly regarded Cochrane Collaboration review criteria for grading the quality of a clinical trial and reviewed 79 RCTs (6462 subjects) that reported on the use of cannabinoids for several medical conditions. In addition to chronic pain, chemotherapy-induced nausea and vomiting (CINV), appetite stimulation in HIV/AIDS, spasticity related to MS or paraplegia, sleep disorders, Tourette syndrome, glaucoma and psychiatric disorders (depression, anxiety and psychosis) were reviewed. The study concluded that the use of cannabinoids appeared to improve symptoms of pain in most of the studies but did not reach statistical significance in a large minority. The authors reported a reduction in chronic pain in eight trials with six studies on neuropathic pain and two trials in cancer. In patients that reported reduction in pain greater than 30%, cannabinoids were superior over placebo. The greatest effect was reported with smoked Δ^9-tetrahydrocannabinol (THC) and the remaining seven trials used nabilone (Whiting et al., 2015).

Clinical Trials of Phytocannabinoids

In many therapeutic areas studies of benefits from cannabinoids are limited and difficult to interpret. Perhaps due to the need to identify non-opioid analgesics and the evolution of social acceptance of cannabis, multiple trials evaluating cannabis in pain are available.

Noncancer pain and neuropathic pain have especially been studied and below is a discussion of several informative trials.

HIV-associated neuropathic pain is the most common neurological complaint of patients with HIV and constitutes approximately 25–50% on visits to pain clinics (Verma, 2001; Dorsey and Morton, 2006). Abrams *et al.* (2007), in a randomized, placebo-controlled study of patients with HIV-associated neuropathic pain treated with smoked cannabis or placebo, found that over half (52%) reported reduction in pain > 30% while 24% of the placebo group reported similar improvement. Patients participating in the study were allowed to take their usual medications including opioids. When patients were challenged with experimentally induced pain from applied heat, no difference was reported between the groups (Abrams *et al.*, 2007).

Neuropathic pain usually is a chronic pain condition that is frequently the result of a progressive disease or injury to the nerve tissue. Chronic neuropathic pain as a result of trauma or surgery was evaluated by Ware *et al.* (2010) utilizing a double-blind, placebo-controlled, four-way crossover design. Patients were allowed to continue their usual pain medications including opioids and most had previous exposure to cannabis. Smoked cannabis containing 25 mg of THC was provided three times a day for five days with a modest but statistically significant reduction in pain intensity reported. Secondary measures of sleep and anxiety were also found to be improved during the cannabis treatment when compared with placebo (Ware *et al.*, 2010).

Abuse and tolerance of cannabinoids would be an obvious concern in treating any chronic condition. Ware *et al.* (2015) evaluated the safety of administering phytocannabinoids for one year in a large, prospective, nonrandomized and nonblinded, multisite study of 431 patients with noncancer chronic pain. Cannabis containing 12.5% THC and 0.5% cannabidiol (CBD) was provided to 216 patients with placebo given to the remaining 215. The patients were allowed to choose their preferred route of administration and to titrate to a maximum dosage up to 5 g/d. The largest group of patients (44%) chose to smoke and ingest cannabinoids, 14% preferred vaporizing, smoking and ingesting, and only 4% elected to only smoke or vaporize cannabis. Safety was determined by the reported number of severe and nonsevere events and secondary outcomes included assessment of neurocognition, pulmonary function and laboratory chemistries.

There was no increase in serious adverse events compared with controls although more nonserious adverse events were reported in the cannabis group. The most common adverse events reported in the cannabis group were CNS (20%) complaints followed by gastrointestinal and pulmonary problems. No change was reported in neurocognitive functions or laboratory renal, liver or endocrine measures. Despite this higher incidence of adverse events, there was a reduction in pain within the cannabis patients but not in the control group. The average dose of cannabis was 2.5 g/d and the authors concluded that the adverse events observed in the study were similar to those encountered with prescription cannabinoids such as nabilone (Lynch and Ware, 2015; Ware *et al.*, 2015).

Clinical Trials of Prescription Cannabinoids

Nabiximols (Sativex)

Nabiximols (Sativex) is a botanical extract containing both THC and CBD and is approved in Canada and Israel. Only in these two countries is nabiximols approved as a prescription medication for neuropathic pain associated with spasticity in MS and for adult patients with advanced cancer who experience moderate to severe pain during the highest tolerated dose of strong opioid therapy for persistent background pain. Although not approved in the USA for any use, nabiximols is available in 28 countries for adjunctive treatment of symptomatic relief of spasticity in adult patients with (MS) who have not responded adequately to other therapies and that demonstrate meaningful improvement during an initial trial of therapy.

Nabiximols may have important benefits in relieving chronic pain from nociceptive and neuropathic etiologies. Several well-conducted trials with nabiximols have evaluated its effect on chronic pain. In one study, 125 patients with peripheral neuropathic pain from various etiologies were randomized in a five-week, double-blind, placebo-controlled, parallel design study. During the study, the patients were allowed to remain on their existing stable analgesic medications and the primary outcome in the study was mean reduction in pain intensity scores. After the addition of nabiximols to their usual use of analgesics, patients were reported to have a greater reduction in pain than those on placebo. Improvements were shown in the secondary outcomes of the Neuropathic Pain Scale (NPS), sleep, dynamic and punctate allodynia, Pain Disability Index (PDI) and Patient Global Impression of Change (PGIC) (Nurmikko et al., 2007).

Brachial plexus root avulsion is a traumatic injury to the nerve with a resultant neuropathic injury. In a second study to evaluate the effectiveness of nabiximols for the treatment of this difficult-to-treat chronic pain, 48 patients with at least one avulsed root enrolled in a randomized, double-blind, placebo-controlled, three-period, crossover study. All patients had intractable symptoms despite treatment with analgesics and most had prior experience with cannabis. After a two-week baseline, patients were then randomized into three, two-week treatment periods during which they received one of three oromucosal spray preparations. The spray treatments were placebo and two different doses of nabiximols. The primary outcome measure was the mean pain severity score during the last seven days of treatment. Secondary outcome measures included pain-related quality of life assessments.

Although the primary outcome failed to achieve the degree of reduction in pain severity hypothesized by the investigators, the difference was still statistically significant along with an associated improvement in sleep. Most of the patients had prior experience with cannabis and the study medications were generally well tolerated with the majority of adverse events reported as mild to moderate in severity (Rog et al., 2005).

Diabetic peripheral neuropathy is the most frequent neuropathy encountered clinically and is associated with considerable pain. Approximately half of patients with diabetes will eventually suffer from the chronic neuropathy (Iqbal et al., 2018) and the usefulness of nabiximols in the long-term treatment of this condition was assessed in an open-label extension study. A total of 380 patients with neuropathy and diabetes or allodynia were enrolled from two previous randomized, controlled trials of nabiximols. Patients were allowed to continue on their analgesics if their dosage was stable and also continue nabiximols for an additional 38 weeks. The daily dose of nabiximols in the two RCTs was similar to the dosing in the extension phase indicating the absence of tolerance to the medication. Neuropathic pain severity was the primary outcome and additional secondary outcomes of sleep quality, NPS scores, subjective global impression of change and EQ-5D questionnaire were collected.

At least half the patients reported a decrease of 30% or greater in the primary outcome of pain severity at all time points in the extension study and the number of patients that reported similar improvement in pain continued to increase over time. Improvements were observed for all secondary efficacy outcomes, and nabiximols was well tolerated for the study duration. Patients did not seek to increase their dose with time and no new safety concerns arose from long-term use. The investigators concluded that nabiximols was useful in the treatment of peripheral neuropathy associated with diabetes or allodynia for most patients (Hoggart et al., 2015).

Cancer pain remains a serious problem frequently inadequately treated with opioids (Gaertner and Schiessl, 2013). Cannabinoids have long been of interest in relieving cancer pain and nabiximols has also been evaluated in several clinical trials. Johnson et al. (2010) reported the effects of nabiximols in 177 patients at multiple European sites with advanced cancer pain that had an inadequate response to opioids. Patients entered a two-week, multicenter, double-blind, randomized, placebo-controlled, parallel-group trial and were randomized to one of three conditions, nabiximols, THC extract and placebo. These were administered using a pump action oromucosal spray. Each actuation of the pump containing nabiximols dosed 2.7 mg THC and 2.5 mg CBD and for the pump containing THC a dose of 2.7 mg THC was delivered. The pump containing placebo delivered only excipients and colorants. The maximum allowed actuations were 8 in any 3-hour period and 48 in any 24-hour period.

Patients could titrate to their preferred dose over the first week. They could increase their dose by 50% each day until they achieved pain relief or encountered side effects. Once the patient had determined the optimal dose, they remained at that level for the duration of the study.

The primary endpoints were the change in pain Numerical Rating Scale (NRS) from baseline and the use of a rescue analgesic. Compared with placebo, nabiximols was statistically better in the change of the mean pain NRS while THC was not statistically different than placebo. There was no change from baseline in median dose of opioid background medication or mean number of doses of breakthrough medication across treatment groups. Forty-three percent of patients randomized to nabiximols reported at least a 30% reduction in pain while the THC and placebo group responses were reported as half this degree of improvement. The authors concluded that nabiximols was superior to THC alone as a useful adjunctive treatment for patients with inadequate analgesic response to opioids (Johnson et al., 2010).

The same authors assessed the possibility of tolerance to the effects of nabiximols in a follow-up study. Forty-three patients with cancer-related pain with mixed etiologies experiencing inadequate analgesia despite chronic opioid dosing and who had participated in the previous three-arm (nabiximols, THC spray or placebo) randomized controlled trial were enrolled in an open-label, multicenter, follow-up study. Twenty-three of these patients had previously been on nabiximols, 11 had been on THC spray, and 19 had received placebo. Titration of the dosing was identical to the earlier trial and nabiximols patients dosed themselves on average 5.4 + 3.28 sprays per day compared with THC spray which was taken on average 14.5 + 16.84 sprays per day.

Although the study was an observational study that sought to determine patient and prescriber behaviors without any formal hypothesis, the Brief Pain Inventory–Short Form (BPI-SF) was used to evaluate potential decrease in pain from baseline to end of study. Most investigators assessed their patient outcomes as "suboptimal" but noted the difficulty in assessing patients with progressive cancer. Significant adverse events were noted in the nabiximols group and included somnolence and confusion (Johnson et al., 2013).

Chemotherapy-induced neuropathic pain (CINP) is another difficult-to-treat pain associated with cancer. In a later study of cancer patients with CINP, Lynch *et al.* (2014) conducted a randomized, placebo-controlled, crossover study in 18 patients treated with nabiximols. Neuropathic pain was measured using an 11-point NRS for pain intensity (NRS-PI), with anchors of "no pain" for the least pain and "pain as bad as you can imagine" for the maximum. The primary outcome measure was change in NRS-PI from baseline (average pain score over seven days pretreatment) to the final week of stable dose treatment. Additional secondary measurements were also obtained and included the Short Form-36 Health Survey (SF-36), quantitative sensory testing (a dynamic allodynia and pinprick assessment), and collection of adverse events. Outcomes were collected at three time points before treatment, at midpoint and the final week of stable dose.

Sixteen patients completed the study and no statistical difference in the numerical rating of pain intensity was noted between groups. Patients randomized to nabiximols used less actuations compared with those taking placebo (8 versus 11) and five patients on nabiximols demonstrated a statistically significant drop in pain intensity. Although the overall study was negative, the authors noted the small sample in this study and the refractory nature of treating chemotherapy-induced neuropathies (Lynch, Cesar-Rittenberg and Hohmann, 2014).

Nabilone and Dronabinol

Nabilone (Cesamet) is a synthetic analog of THC and dronabinol (Marinol and Syndros) is THC made through a chemical synthesis without any plant-based constituents. Although both have been available for prescription use since the mid-1980s neither are approved for use as an analgesic. However, as cannabinoids available for prescription, they have been of interest as a potential treatment for chronic pain.

Nabilone is currently approved in several countries including the USA and Canada and in the EU for CINV. Berlach *et al.* (2006), first studied 20 patients with mixed noncancer etiologies for chronic pain who were treated with nabilone in a small clinical trial. Fifteen of the 20 subjects reported improvement of pain and 9 also reported a reduction in pain intensity. These patients had previously been treated with standard analgesics and a small majority had used cannabis (Berlach, Shir and Ware, 2006).

Diabetic peripheral neuropathic pain (DPN) is another chronic neuropathic condition that has been treated with nabilone. In a randomized, double-blind, placebo-controlled, enriched study Toth *et al.* (2012) studied 37 patients with well-diagnosed treatment-resistant DPN. Patients were initially enrolled in a single-blind, flexible dose lead-in study with nabilone for four weeks. During the first week patients were dosed with nabilone 0.5 mg BID and titrated upward to a maximum dose of 2 mg BID as tolerated over the subsequent three weeks. At the end of the fourth week, 26 patients (out of 35) reported > 30% pain relief on a steady dose of nabilone during the final seven days and were eligible to enroll in the second phase of the study.

The second phase was a five-week, randomized, double-blind comparison study of nabilone versus placebo in DPN. Patients were randomized to continue their mean dose of nabilone that had been determined over the last seven days of the lead-in phase or to receive placebo. If placed on placebo, the patients were titrated off their previous nabilone dose within the first week. The primary outcome was the mean daily pain score over the last seven days of the second phase of the study compared with the mean daily pain score during baseline. Secondary measures were also collected and similarly compared.

Nabilone was found to be statistically better than placebo in the reduction of pain. The majority of nabilone-treated patients (11 out of 13) reported reduction in daily pain and a minority (4 out of 13) reported > 50% reduction. In contrast, only five patients randomized to placebo in the second phase continued to report reduction in pain from baseline.

Three secondary measures were also statistically significant in the nabilone-treated group. Improvement in sleep measured by the Medical Outcomes Sleep Survey (MOSS), reduction in the anxiety subscale of the Hospital Anxiety and Depression Scale (HADS), and European Quality of Life-5-Domains were all significantly improved compared with baseline scores. The authors concluded that nabilone is a useful adjunctive treatment in patients with DPN although the mechanism of action through cannabinoid receptors or non-cannabinoid receptors has yet to be determined (Toth *et al.*, 2012).

Dronabinol has also been studied in patients with central neuropathic pain associated with MS in a randomized, double-blind, placebo-controlled, crossover trial. Twenty-four patients between the ages of 23 and 55 years were enrolled. Unlike many of the clinical trials evaluating cannabinoids, in this study the investigators restricted the use of concomitant analgesic medications with the exception of paracetamol at least one week before the first visit. Either dronabinol up to a maximum dose of 10 mg/d or placebo was administered to the patients for three weeks. Patients then entered a three-week washout before starting on the alternate condition. The primary outcome measurement was the median spontaneous pain intensity in the last week of each treatment. Secondary outcome measurements collected were median radiating pain intensity in the last week of treatment, pain relief, use of escape medication, patient preference, health-related quality of life (SF-36), Expanded Disability Status Scale (EDSS) score and quantitative sensory testing.

The primary outcome of median spontaneous pain intensity was significantly lower during the dronabinol treatment compared with placebo. The difference between dronabinol and placebo in reduction of pain was approximately 21%. On the secondary measures, two items on the SF-36 quality of life scale, bodily pain and mental health, demonstrated improvement with dronabinol over placebo. Adverse events including dizziness occurred most frequently in the first week of treatment with dronabinol. The authors concluded that dronabinol has a modest but clinically relevant analgesic effect on central pain in patients with MS (Svendsen, Jensen and Bach, 2004).

Neuroprotection is another possible property of cannabinoids in neurodegenerative disorders such as Alzheimer's disease and MS. Zajicek *et al.* (2013) evaluated whether dronabinol could be neuroprotective in a three-year trial of patients with MS. Patients with primary or secondary progressive MS were recruited in this multicenter, parallel, randomized, double-blind, placebo-controlled study and were randomly assigned to receive either dronabinol or placebo. The primary outcomes were the EDSS progression of at least one point from the baseline score or 0.5 point from an EDSS score of 5.5, and change from baseline in the physical impact subscale of the 29-item Multiple Sclerosis Impact Scale (MSIS-29-PHYS).

A total of 498 patients were randomized and received at least one dose of dronabinol and 145 patients received at least one dose of placebo. A four-week titration period was included for both groups with initial doses at 3.5 mg dronabinol BID that were titrated up to a maximum of 28 mg/d upon patient bodyweight and tolerability.

No statistical differences in slowing down the progression of disease were reported between the dronabinol group and placebo. There are several factors that may contribute to the failure to find delays in progression of MS with dronabinol. Although patients could remain in this study for three years, many patients discontinued especially those treated with dronabinol due to side effects. Retention of patients in any long-term studies is difficult and in this study the adverse events related to dronabinol may have been contributory (Zajicek *et al.*, 2013).

There has been extensive interest over the past several years that cannabinoids may reduce the dosage of opioids in certain pain conditions. Narang *et al.* (2008) examined this potential effect of dronabinol as an adjunctive treatment in patients taking opioids for chronic, noncancer pain. The study evaluated patients with various etiologies for chronic pain and was divided into two phases. Phase one was a single-dose, double-blinded, randomized, crossover, placebo-controlled study and was followed by a phase two, open-label, multidose extension.

In the first phase of the study, 47 patients continued their usual opioid medication and were randomized to three conditions that consisted of either 10 mg or 20 mg of dronabinol or placebo. After the first treatment they were then crossed over to receive the other two conditions separated by at least three days. The primary outcome was total pain relief at 8 hours (TOTPAR) after medication administration. Additional measurements collected during the clinic visit included baseline self-report, hourly ratings of pain intensity, pain relief, treatment satisfaction, pain bothersomeness, mood, side effects, and blood serum levels were obtained.

Thirty patients elected to continue into the four-week, open-label extension trial of dronabinol as an adjunctive medication to stable doses of opioids. Dronabinol initially was administered at 5 mg BID and then titrated by the patient for optimal results. The minimal dose of dronabinol could be as low as 5 mg daily and maximum was up to 20 mg TID. Patients were permitted to increase the dronabinol after being on their dose for two days or to reduce it at any time for side effects. However, they were instructed to maintain a stable dose of dronabinol during the final week of the study. Patients could decide at any time to reduce their opioids during the second phase.

For the second phase, the primary outcome was change in pain intensity from baseline measured by a numeric scale. For both phases of the study secondary measurements included patient satisfaction, side effects, dropout rate, adverse events, mood and pain bothersomeness. In addition, five questionnaires were administered during the first visit of the initial phase of the study and during the final visit of the second phase of the study: BPI-SF, HADS, Symptom Checklist, RAND 36-Item Health Survey, and the Medical Outcomes Study Sleep (MOSS) scale.

The results from the first phase study showed that patients who received dronabinol experienced decreased pain intensity and increased satisfaction compared with those receiving placebo. No differences in benefit were found between the 10 mg and 20 mg doses. In the second phase, titrated dronabinol contributed to a statistically significant relief of pain, reduced pain bothersomeness and increased satisfaction compared with baseline. The incidence of side effects was dose related. The authors concluded that the use of dronabinol resulted in additional analgesia among patients taking opioids for chronic noncancer pain despite taking stable doses of opioids (Narang *et al.*, 2008).

Finally, a recent meta-analysis of chronic pain with neuropathic components of various etiologies treated with cannabinoids was published by Mücke *et al.* (2018). In this study, the author selected from the published literature randomized, double-blind controlled clinical trials of medical cannabis, plant-derived or synthetic cannabis-based medications against placebo or active treatments. The study had to include at least 10 patients and have a duration of at least two weeks. Sixteen studies were identified involving 1750 people and lasting between 2 and 26 weeks. Ten studies compared combinations of THC and CBD, two studies compared nabilone, two studies were found with inhaled herbal cannabis and two studies with dronabinol. Fifteen studies were placebo-controlled and one compared nabilone with dihydrocodeine.

From this analysis of mixed data, the authors concluded there was no high-level evidence that cannabinoids are effective in neuropathic pain. However, cannabis-based medicines when pooled together were better than placebo in reducing pain intensity, sleep problems and psychological distress. Surprisingly, herbal cannabis when analyzed without the prescription cannabinoids was not different from placebo in reducing pain and the number of people who dropped out due to side effects (very low-quality evidence) (Mücke *et al.*, 2018).

Cannabinoids in Cancer Pain

Earlier in this chapter nabiximols was reviewed and the absence of approval in the USA was noted. Despite approval in 28 countries for neuropathic pain associated with spasticity in MS, in only Canada and Israel is it approved for adult patients with advanced cancer who experience moderate to severe pain during the highest tolerated dose of strong opioid therapy for persistent background pain. In the USA three large-scale studies evaluating nabiximols as adjunctive therapy in advanced cancer patients were conducted by GW Pharma and Otsuka Pharmaceuticals as the US development partner. All three phase III studies failed to show superiority over placebo (Fallon *et al.*, 2017; Lichtman *et al.*, 2018).

Fallon *et al.* (2017) was the first to report the failure of two phase III studies. Both studies were similar double-blind, randomized, placebo-controlled trials with the same primary outcome and patient eligibility and study criteria. In one study, however, only patients that had shown improvement treated with reduction of pain were allowed to be randomized to the study drug versus placebo condition. Despite including this enriched population of responders, both studies failed to show superiority of nabiximols over placebo in the cancer population (Fallon *et al.*, 2017)

Lichtman *et al.* (2018) reported on the final of the three phase III studies. The study was a double-blind, randomized, placebo-controlled trial in patients with advanced cancer and chronic pain uncontrolled by optimized opioid therapy. Patients were randomized to nabiximols (199) or placebo (198) and allowed to titrate the study medications over a two-week period. Once the optimal dose had been established, the patient continued on the fixed dose for three weeks. The study primary endpoint was percent improvement from baseline to end of treatment in average pain NRS scores. The study reported the median percent improvements from baseline to end of treatment in the nabiximols and placebo groups were 10.7% vs. 4.5% ($p = 0.0854$) (Lichtman *et al.*, 2018).

Cannabinoid–Opiate Interactions

In Chapter 1 the birth of the modern pharmaceutical industry was introduced and attributed to the chemical separation of the analgesic morphine from the opium plant between 1803 and 1805 by the German pharmacologist Friedrich Sertürner. From the beginning, development of analgesics has been the subject of considerable pharmaceutical development yet better treatments remain desperately needed.

Cannabinoids have also been used as analgesics throughout history but, unlike morphine, only in the last 50 years have cannabinoids been isolated from the plant *Cannabis sativa*. Once cannabinoids were chemically isolated the properties of the endocannabinoid system (ECS) could be determined. This research has led to the recognition that the ECS is a second system that perceives and responds to pain.

There is a significant amount of preclinical data to support the belief that cannabinoids and opiates interact with each other and may be complementary systems. In animal studies, it is well established that the nociceptive pathways that sense and communicate pain are shared by overlapping distributions of cannabinoid and opiate receptors. In the dorsal horn of the spinal cord, CB_1 receptors and the opiate μ receptors overlap and together modulate nociceptive signaling at the spinal cord level, and in the periaqueductal gray area (PAG), the raphe and the thalamic nuclei both receptors are abundantly expressed. In addition, both are positioned on the presynaptic membrane of neurons and are G protein-coupled receptors that inhibit calcium channel flows and activate potassium.

There are other functions shared by both systems. For instance, both cannabinoid and opiate receptor agonists block both nociceptive and neuropathic pain in preclinical studies. Finally, cannabinoids and opiate receptors share other physiological processes including hypothermia, hypotension, sedation-reduced locomotor activity and gastrointestinal motility.

In 2014 Bachhuber *et al.* (2014) published a widely referenced report suggesting that death by opioid overdose was reduced in states that had legalized the use of cannabis. Reviewing deaths by opioid overdose between 1998 and 2010, the authors estimated a 24.8% reduction in expected overdose deaths per 100,000 in states that legalized medical cannabis (Bachhuber *et al.*, 2014).

This intriguing observation that cannabis somehow reduced the need for opioids or protected against the lethal overdose was followed by several epidemiological studies that provided further support that the relationship between the opiate and cannabinoid systems may be beneficial. One time series analysis reported a 6% decrease in two years of opiate-related deaths following the legalization of cannabis in Colorado (Livingston *et al.*, 2017). This implied a reduction in opiate use or dosage. In a second retrospective study of prospective medication claims for opiates to Medicare and Medicaid plans, states that legalized marijuana reported fewer doses of prescribed opiates when compared with states that had limited access (Bradford and Bradford, 2017). A further publication by the same authors found a reduction in opioid prescriptions in states with marijuana dispensaries. In this longitudinal analysis a statistical decline in prescriptions for hydrocodone was reported with a numerical decline for fentanyl (Bradford and Bradford, 2017). Similarly, in another study, analysis of Medicaid prescription data showed a reduction in opiate use of 5.88% in states with legalized medical cannabis use and 6.38% reduction when recreational cannabis was also permitted (Wen and Hockenberry, 2018). Other large-scale observational studies of cannabis use have also been published (Haroutounian *et al.*, 2016). Collectively, these surveys suggest that patients with chronic nociceptive or neuropathic pain may have better analgesic benefits when using cannabis with opiates.

As interesting as these results are reporting reduction in opioid prescriptions and fewer deaths by overdose, a recent study by Shover *et al.* (2019) did not replicate the findings of reduced mortality. The data reported by Bachhuber *et al.* (2014) was reanalyzed and extended to a longer period of time (1999–2017). In this analysis of a larger pool of data, states legalizing medical cannabis had a 22.7% increase in overdose deaths. The authors speculated that the original finding that reported a causal relationship between medical cannabis and a reduction in opioid overdoses was not supported by the larger analysis and that no positive association could be found between permissive medical cannabis laws and opioid overdose mortality. Instead, they suggested that other factors yet to be identified were influential in overdose fatalities (Shover et al., 2019).

Although cannabinoids are extremely safe with respect to overdose, long-term use has been associated with drug dependence. In a population already at great risk for addiction using opiates, exposing these same patients to the added potential of cannabis dependence needs to be carefully considered. In the past there was controversy regarding the addictive potential of cannabinoids but cannabis use disorder (CUD) is now recognized as a clinical issue in DSM-5. Like many addictive drugs, higher doses and longer durations of use carry greater risk of addiction. The increasing potency of cannabinoids with longer duration of exposure for chronic problems in these populations only add to these concerns.

In a large, retrospective study of patients in the US Veterans Affairs system, those patients receiving opiates for noncancer pain were found to have increased opiate refills if they also had CUD (Hefner, Sofuoglu and Rosenheck, 2015). Those patients diagnosed with CUD that received approved prescriptions for opiates were more likely to also present with other mental disorders including schizophrenia and bipolar disease, physical illness including hepatic disease or HIV in addition to dependence on other substances including alcohol, stimulants and tobacco. This study examined the medical records of 1,316,464 veterans with noncancer pain diagnoses that received opioid medications in fiscal year 2012. Although the study was limited in that only semi-structured interviews of a homogeneous male-predominant population were conducted, the authors advised that the risk of CUD and coadministration of cannabis and opiates requires further study (Hefner, Sofuoglu and Rosenheck, 2015).

There are several small clinical studies that suggest that cannabis can enhance the analgesic effects of opioids. In one study by Cooper et al. (2018), the analgesic effect of a very low dose of oxycodone in combination with cannabis was investigated. In this study, 18 "healthy" cannabis users were given an ultra-small dose of oxycodone (2.5 mg PO) with either smoked placebo cannabis (THC = 0%) or active smoked cannabis (THC = 5.6%). Although these participants were healthy and did not have pain complaints, pain was experimentally induced by instructing them to place their hands in ice water (cold pressor test) until they could not tolerate the procedure. Significant reduction in pain was found with active cannabis and low-dose oxycodone in combination although no analgesic effect was reported with active cannabis alone or low-dose oxycodone alone.

In addition to demonstrating a synergistic effect between cannabinoids and opiates, an important question on the safety included abuse liability and needed to be addressed. The combination did not increase the abuse liability for cannabis and participants did not increase the self-administration of cannabis. The use of oxycodone also did not increase with the likability of cannabis. However, when used in combination, the participants reported a small increase in 'liking' oxycodone with a higher abuse likability rating.

The study was unable to evaluate whether self-administration of the opiate would increase in tandem with the greater abuse liability. This would be an important question to answer in future studies especially in chronic patients where they are exposed to opiates and cannabis for a prolonged duration (Cooper et al., 2018).

Although the preclinical studies, small clinical trials and epidemiological studies are suggestive that cannabinoids and opioids interact, firm conclusions are not yet established. A recent meta-analysis of clinical trials that reviewed the existing information on reduction of opiate dosage with coadministration of cannabinoids found only limited clinical support with no strong conclusions (Nielsen *et al.*, 2017).

Headache and Migraine

William O'Shaughnessy is frequently credited with introducing cannabis to western medicine as a remedy for headache in 1839 when he presented his observations to the medical colleagues at the Medical College of Calcutta (Booth, 2004). Interest in the analgesic effects of cannabis became widely accepted in the practice of medicine and many prominent doctors touted its benefits. Sir William Osler, recognized with the accolade "father of modern medicine," once wrote that "one of the first duties of the physician is to advise the masses not to take any medicines" and is considered by many "a therapeutic nihilist" (Ryan, 2019). Yet he recommended in his influential 1892 textbook *The Principles and Practice of Medicine* the use of cannabis as both an acute and maintenance treatment for migraine (Boes, 2015). In the *United States Pharmacopeia*, a national formulary, cannabis was listed as a drug to treat numerous ailments including headache and migraine throughout the nineteenth century and the first part of the twentieth century. Only in 1941 were cannabis preparations removed from the pharmacopeia after federal legislation banned the sale of cannabis in the United States (Booth, 2004).

Despite this historic recognition of cannabinoids as useful medications for headache and migraine, it is surprising that the supporting evidence is limited to case-based, anecdotal or laboratory-based scientific research (Baron, 2018). As discussed earlier in this chapter, CB_1 and CB_2 receptors are richly expressed in areas associated with pain including the dorsal horn of the spinal cord, the PAG, rostral medulla, and thalamus. In addition, the nucleus trigeminal caudalis and ganglia (Greco *et al.*, 2010; McGeeney, 2013) have been identified as associated with migraine and are rich in CB_1 receptors. The PAG, an area within the tegmentum of the midbrain, has strong associations with the origination of migraine and functions as the control center for descending pain messaging. CB_1 receptors are plentiful in the PAG and activation is believed to modulate nociceptive input from the trigeminal ganglion.

Russo (2016) has suggested that migraine may be an endocannabinoid deficiency and levels of the endocannabinoid *N*-arachidonoylethanolamide (anandamide; AEA) in the cerebrospinal fluid have been reported to be reduced in patients with migraine (Sarchielli *et al.*, 2007). In addition, fatty acid amide hydrolase (FAAH), the principal enzyme that breaks down AEA, has been reported to be reduced in chronic migraine and medication overuse headache compared with controls (Cupini *et al.*, 2008; Rossi *et al.*, 2008). The same group also reported increased activity of FAAH in females but not males with episodic migraine (Cupini *et al.*, 2006; Greco *et al.*, 2018).

As discussed in previous chapters, both endocannabinoids and phytocannabinoids assert their pharmacological effects through CB_1 and CB_2 receptors and through multiple non-cannabinoid receptor targets that bind AEA. Among these, the TRPV family of receptors found in the trigeminal ganglion are major targets for AEA. In addition, AEA has also been found to influence serotonin, known to be involved in headache, through potentiation of $5HT_{1A}$ receptor responses and inhibition of $5HT_{2A}$ and $5HT_3$ receptor responses.

Although there is a paucity of controlled studies of cannabis in the treatment of headache and migraine (McGeeney, 2013), there are a few single-case reports reporting benefits from smoked cannabis or oral dronabinol. One retrospective study of 121 adults with the diagnosis of migraine treated with medical cannabis at a medical cannabis clinic found a significant drop in the frequency of headache. However, pain is highly subjective and influenced by many physical and psychological variables. Understanding the benefit of cannabis in open retrospective chart review is difficult to determine and much additional work needs to be done (Rhyne *et al.*, 2016).

Bibliography

Abrams, D. I. *et al.* (2007) 'Cannabis in painful HIV-associated sensory neuropathy: a randomized placebo-controlled trial', *Neurology*, 68(7), 515–521. doi:10.1212/01. wnl.0000253187.66183.9 c.

Aviram, J. and Samuelly-Leichtag, G. (2017) 'Efficacy of cannabis-based medicines for pain management: a systematic review and meta-analysis of randomized controlled trials', *Pain Physician*, 20(6), E755–E796.

Bachhuber, M. A. *et al.* (2014) 'Medical cannabis laws and opioid analgesic overdose mortality in the United States, 1999-2010', *JAMA Internal Medicine*, 174(10), 1668–1673. doi:10.1001/jamainternmed.2014.4005.

Baron, E. P. (2018) 'Medicinal properties of cannabinoids, terpenes, and flavonoids in cannabis, and benefits in migraine, headache, and pain: an update on current evidence and cannabis science', *Headache*, 58(7), 1139–1186. doi:10.1111/head.13345.

Berlach, D. M., Shir, Y. and Ware, M. A. (2006) 'Experience with the synthetic cannabinoid nabilone in chronic noncancer pain', *Pain Medicine*, 7(1), pp. 25–29. doi:10.1111/j.1526-4637.2006.00085.x.

Boehnke, K. A. *et al.* (2019) 'Qualifying conditions of medical cannabis license holders in the United States', *Health Affairs*, 38(2), 295–302. doi:10.1377/hlthaff.2018.05266.

Boes, C. J. (2015) 'Osler on migraine', *Canadian Journal of Neurological Sciences*, 42(2), 144–147. https://doi.org/10.1017/cjn.2015.6.

Booth, M. (2004) *Cannabis: A History.* New York: St. Martin's Press.

Bradford, A. C. and Bradford, W. D. (2017) 'Medical marijuana laws may be associated with a decline in the number of prescriptions for medicaid enrollees', *Health Affairs*, 36(5), 945–951. doi:10.1377/hlthaff.2016.1135.

Cooper, Z. *et al.* (2018) 'Impact of co-administration of oxycodone and smoked cannabis on analgesia and abuse liability', *Neuropsychopharmacology*, 43, 2046–2018. doi:10.1038/s41386-018-0011-2.

Cupini, L. M. *et al.* (2006) 'Biochemical changes in endocannabinoid system are expressed in platelets of female but not male migraineurs', *Cephalalgia*, 26(3), 277–281. doi:10.1111/j.1468-2982.2005.01031.x.

Cupini, L. M. *et al.* (2008) 'Degradation of endocannabinoids in chronic migraine and medication overuse headache', *Neurobiology of Disease*, 30(2), 186–189. doi:10.1016/j.nbd.2008.01.003.

Dorsey, S. G. and Morton, P. G. (2006) 'HIV peripheral neuropathy: pathophysiology and clinical implications', *AACN Advanced Critical Care*, 17(1), 30–36. doi:10.1097/00044067-200601000-00004.

Fallon, M. T. *et al.* (2017) 'Sativex oromucosal spray as adjunctive therapy in advanced cancer patients with chronic pain unalleviated by optimized opioid therapy: two double-blind, randomized, placebo-controlled phase 3 studies', *British Journal of Pain*, 11(3), 119–133. doi:10.1177/2049463717710042.

Finniss, D. G. *et al.* (2010) 'Biological, clinical, and ethical advances of placebo effects', *The Lancet*, 375(9715), 686–695. doi:10.1016/S0140-6736(09)61706-2.

Gaertner, J. and Schiessl, C. (2013) 'Cancer pain management: what's new?', *Current Pain and Headache Reports*, 17(4), 328. doi:10.1007/s11916-013-0328-9.

Greco, R. *et al.* (2010) 'The endocannabinoid system and migraine', *Experimental Neurology*, 224(1), 85–91. doi:10.1016/j.expneurol.2010.03.029.

Greco, R. *et al.* (2018) 'Endocannabinoid system and migraine pain: an update', *Frontiers in Neuroscience*, 12,172. doi:10.3389/fnins.2018.00172.

Haroutounian, S. *et al.* (2016) 'The effect of medicinal cannabis on pain and quality-of-life outcomes in chronic pain: a prospective open-label study', *Clinical Journal of Pain*, 32(12), 1036–1043. doi:10.1097/AJP.0000000000000364.

Hefner, K., Sofuoglu, M. and Rosenheck, R. (2015) 'Concomitant cannabis abuse/dependence in patients treated with opioids for non-cancer pain', *American Journal of Addiction*, 24(6), 538–545. doi:10.1111/ajad.12260.

Hoggart, B. *et al.* (2015) 'A multicentre, open-label, follow-on study to assess the long-term maintenance of effect, tolerance and safety of THC/CBD oromucosal spray in the management of neuropathic pain', *Journal of Neurology*, 262(1), 27–40. doi:10.1007/s00415-014-7502-9.

Iqbal, Z. *et al.* (2018) 'Diabetic peripheral neuropathy: epidemiology, diagnosis, and pharmacotherapy', *Clinical Therapeutics*, 40(6), 828–849. doi:10.1016/j.clinthera.2018.04.001.

Johnson, J. R. *et al.* (2010) 'Multicenter, double-blind, randomized, placebo-controlled, parallel-group study of the efficacy, safety, and tolerability of THC:CBD extract and THC extract in patients with intractable cancer-related pain', *Journal of Pain and Symptom Management*, 39(2), 167–179. doi:10.1016/j.jpainsymman.2009.06.008.

Johnson, J. R. *et al.* (2013) 'An open-label extension study to investigate the long-term safety and tolerability of THC/CBD oromucosal spray and oromucosal THC spray in patients with terminal

cancer-related pain refractory to strong opioid analgesics', *Journal of Pain and Symptom Management*, 46(2), 207–218. doi:10.1016/j.jpainsymman.2012.07.014.

Lichtman, A. H. *et al.* (2018) 'Results of a double-blind, randomized, placebo-controlled study of nabiximols oromucosal spray as an adjunctive therapy in advanced cancer patients with chronic uncontrolled pain', *Journal of Pain and Symptom Management*, 55(2), 179.e1–188.e1. doi:10.1016/j.jpainsymman.2017.09.001.

Livingston, M. D. *et al.* (2017) 'Recreational cannabis legalization and opioid-related deaths in Colorado, 2000-2015', *American Journal of Public Health*, 107(11), 1827–1829. doi:10.2105/AJPH.2017.304059.

Lynch, M. E., Cesar-Rittenberg, P. and Hohmann, A. G. (2014) 'A double-blind, placebo-controlled, crossover pilot trial with extension using an oral mucosal cannabinoid extract for treatment of chemotherapy-induced neuropathic pain', *Journal of Pain and Symptom Management*, 47(1), 166–173. doi:10.1016/j.jpainsymman.2013.02.018.

Lynch, M. E. and Ware, M. A. (2015) 'Cannabinoids for the treatment of chronic non-cancer pain: an updated systematic review of randomized controlled trials', *Journal of Neuroimmune Pharmacology*, 10(2), 293–301. doi:10.1007/s11481-015-9600-6.

McGeeney, B. E. (2013) 'Cannabinoids and hallucinogens for headache', *Headache*, 53(3), 447–458. doi:10.1111/head.12025.

Mücke, M. *et al.* (2018) 'Cannabis-based medicines for chronic neuropathic pain in adults', *Cochrane Database of Systematic Reviews*, 3, CD012182. doi:10.1002/14651858.CD012182.pub2.

Narang, S. *et al.* (2008) 'Efficacy of dronabinol as an adjuvant treatment for chronic pain patients on opioid therapy', *The Journal of Pain*, 9(3), 254–264. doi:10.1016/j.jpain.2007.10.018.

Nestler, E., Hyman, S. E. and Malenka, R. C. (eds.) (2001) *Molecular Neuropharmacology*. New York: McGraw-Hill.

Nielsen, S. *et al.* (2017) 'Opioid-sparing effect of cannabinoids: a systematic review and meta-analysis', *Neuropsychopharmacology*, 42(9), 1752–1765. doi:10.1038/npp.2017.51.

Nurmikko, T. J. *et al.* (2007) 'Sativex successfully treats neuropathic pain characterised by allodynia: a randomised, double-blind, placebo-controlled clinical trial', *Pain*, 133 (1–3), 210–220. doi:10.1016/j. pain.2007.08.028.

Reynolds, J. R. (1890) 'On the therapeutical uses and toxic effects of Cannabis indica', *The Lancet*, 135(3473), 637–638. doi:10.1016/S0140-6736(02)18723-X.

Rhyne, D. N. *et al.* (2016) 'Effects of medical marijuana on migraine headache frequency in an adult population', *Pharmacotherapy*, 36 (5), 505–510. doi:10.1002/phar.1673.

Rog, D. J. *et al.* (2005) 'Randomized, controlled trial of cannabis-based medicine in central pain in multiple sclerosis', *Neurology*, 65(6), 812–819. doi:10.1212/01. wnl.0000176753.45410.8b.

Rossi, C. *et al.* (2008) 'Endocannabinoids in platelets of chronic migraine patients and medication-overuse headache patients: relation with serotonin levels', *European Journal of Clinical Pharmacology*, 64(1), 1–8. doi:10.1007/s00228-007-0391-4.

Russo, E. B. (2016) 'Clinical endocannabinoid deficiency reconsidered: current research supports the theory in migraine, fibromyalgia, irritable bowel, and other treatment-resistant syndromes', *Cannabis and Cannabinoid Research*, 1(1), 154–165. doi:10.1089/can.2016.0009.

Ryan, T. (2019) 'Osler Centenary Papers: Osler the clinician and scientist: a personal and historical perspective', *Postgraduate Medical Journal*, 95(1130), 660–663. doi:10.1136/postgradmedj-2019-136645.

Sarchielli, P. *et al.* (2007) 'Endocannabinoids in chronic migraine: CSF findings suggest a system failure', *Neuropsychopharmacology*, 32(6), 1384–1390. doi:10.1038/sj. npp.1301246.

Shover, C. L. *et al.* (2019) 'Association between medical cannabis laws and opioid overdose mortality has reversed over time', *Proceedings*

of the National Academy of Sciences of the United States of America, 116(26), 12624–12626. doi:10.1073/pnas.1903434116.

Svendsen, K. B., Jensen, T. S. and Bach, F. W. (2004) 'Does the cannabinoid dronabinol reduce central pain in multiple sclerosis? Randomised double blind placebo controlled crossover trial', *BMJ*, 329(7460), 253. doi:10.1136/bmj.38149.566979.AE.

Toth, C. *et al.* (2012) 'An enriched-enrolment, randomized withdrawal, flexible-dose, double-blind, placebo-controlled, parallel assignment efficacy study of nabilone as adjuvant in the treatment of diabetic peripheral neuropathic pain', *Pain*, 153(10), 2073–2082. doi:10.1016/j.pain.2012.06.024.

Verma, A. (2001) 'Epidemiology and clinical features of HIV-1 associated neuropathies', *Journal of the Peripheral Nervous System*, 6 (1), 8–13. doi:10.1046/j.1529-8027.2001.006001008.x.

Ware, M. A. *et al.* (2010) 'Smoked cannabis for chronic neuropathic pain: a randomized controlled trial', *CMAJ*, 182(14), E694–E701. doi:10.1503/cmaj.091414.

Ware, M. A. *et al.* (2015) 'Cannabis for the Management of Pain: Assessment of Safety Study (COMPASS)', *The Journal of Pain*, 16 (12), 1233–1242. doi:10.1016/j. jpain.2015.07.014.

Wen, H. and Hockenberry, J. M. (2018) 'Association of medical and adult-use marijuana laws with opioid prescribing for medicaid enrollees', *JAMA Internal Medicine*, 178(5), 673–679. doi:10.1001/jamainternmed.2018.1007.

Whiting, P. F. *et al.* (2015) 'Cannabinoids for medical use: a systematic review and meta-analysis', *JAMA: Journal of the American Medical Association*, 313(24), 2456–2473. doi:10.1001/jama.2015.6358.

Zajicek, J. *et al.* (2013) 'Effect of dronabinol on progression in progressive multiple sclerosis (CUPID): a randomised, placebo-controlled trial', *The Lancet Neurology*, 12(9), 857–865. doi:10.1016/S1474-4422(13)70159-5.

Cannabinoids and Neuropsychiatry

I saw in hashish . . . a significant means of exploring the genesis of mental illness . . . It could solve the enigma of mental illness and lead to the hidden source of the mysterious disorder we call "madness" . . .

Jacques-Joseph Moreau, Du Hachisch Et De L'aliénation Mentale: Études Psychologiques

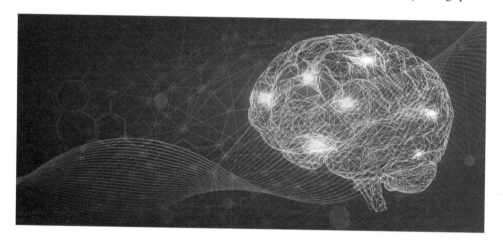

- Activation of the CB_1 (and perhaps the CB_2) receptor may reduce anxiety.
- There is limited evidence in small clinical trials that cannabidiol (CBD) may reduce anxiety.
- CB_1 blockade by the anti-obesity drug rimonabant resulted in severe depression and suicidal ideation.
- Plasma *N*-arachidonoylethanolamide (anandamide; AEA) and 2-arachidonoylglycerol (2-AG) were found to be reduced in depressed women when compared with controls in one study.
- The literature regarding CBD as an antidepressant is inconclusive in a recent (2020) meta-analysis.
- A greater expression of CB_1 receptors in the dorsal lateral prefrontal cortex (DLPFC) was found in postmortem analysis of brains in successful depressed suicide individuals.
- AEA was found to be elevated in the cerebrospinal fluid of patients with schizophrenia.
- The CB_1 expression may be increased in patients with schizophrenia. In an in vivo PET study of 67 patients increased levels of the receptor were found in the cingulate and insular cortex. Postmortem studies, however, have been inconclusive.

Jacques-Joseph Moreau was a French psychiatrist in the nineteenth century and an early contributor to the field of psychopharmacology. During a trip in the 1830s to Egypt to study medical customs in the Middle East, Moreau was introduced to hashish, a dried resin from the marijuana flower, as a treatment for both physical and behavioral ailments.

Upon his return to France in 1839, Moreau began to experiment with several of the psychoactive herbs he had been introduced to including hashish. Moreau believed understanding the psychoactive effects of hashish could serve as a window into the origins of mental disease. In 1845, he published *Du Hachisch Et De L'aliénation Mentale: Études Psychologiques* (translated as *Hashish and Mental Illness* in 1973) and introduced his observations about the hashish-induced psychosis he observed in his patients and also through self-administration. Moreau proposed that hallucinations were fundamental to understanding the origin of mental disorders. Hallucinations, rather than being due to lesions in the brain resulting in structural causes of behavioral changes, were breakdowns between the sensory perception of wakefulness and the dreaming in sleep that led to mental illness.

Modern psychopharmacology has progressed far from these early observations by Moreau. Unexpected outcomes during the treatment of patients by watchful clinicians remain today an important approach to advance our knowledge of mental illness (Klein, 2008). The many properties of the endocannabinoid system (ECS) including the well-established psychoactive effects of Δ^9-tetrahydrocannabinol (THC) make cannabinoids a promising area for observation and future discoveries in neuropsychiatry.

In this chapter we will review selected preclinical and clinical studies that may lead to further development of cannabinoids as treatment for neuropsychiatric disease. Unlike other promising therapeutic areas of medicine where cannabinoids might one day be used, only five cannabinoid-based products are available as prescription medicine and all influence central nervous system (CNS) functions. As previously reviewed in Chapter 4, the US Food and Drug Administration (FDA), Canada Health, the European Medicines Agency (EMA) and other countries in Asia, Australia and Latin America have approved indications. As approved medications, they are available for doctors to prescribe to their patients today. Surprisingly, as a group, cannabinoid-based medicines are not widely used as a result of poor tolerability and efficacy, although promise remains for treatment of other CNS diseases including neurodegenerative diseases such as Parkinson's disease and amyotrophic lateral sclerosis (ALS), Alzheimer's disease, stroke, schizophrenia, depression and anxiety. Our knowledge is incomplete, clinical trials are small and limited in number, and much still remains to be accomplished.

In the absence of high-quality, adequately sized and randomized clinical trials, medical marijuana has not yet met the standard to be approved as a prescription drug. Despite this gap in medical knowledge and approved products, however, there remains a pressing clinical need to treat many neuropsychiatric diseases. In the absence of medicines with known safety and efficacy, medical marijuana has been heavily promoted as treatments for these inadequately treated conditions. For the clinician, weighing the potential benefits and risks of using products that are inadequately studied, the safety of the patient should always be the first concern. Although the emerging science of cannabinoids is intriguing, any recommendations for treatment when our knowledge remains incomplete should be made with careful thought.

Neuropsychiatry and the Endocannabinoid System (ECS)

As discussed in Chapter 3, the ECS consists of at least two endocannabinoids, 2-arachidonoylglycerol (2-AG) and N-arachidonoylethanolamide, also known as anandamide (AEA), two identified cannabinoid receptors (CB_1 and CB_2) and various enzymes that are involved in the synthesis and breakdown of the endocannabinoids. Although the CB_1 receptor is found in multiple organs of the body including the heart, lungs, gastrointestinal tract, eyes, skin and endocrine glands, this receptor is also densely expressed on neurons within the CNS. In comparison, the CB_2 receptor is found extensively in the lymphatic and peripheral immune system with a limited presence in the CNS where it can be found in the cerebellum and activated glial cells.

Within the brain, the cannabinoid receptors (especially CB_1) are abundantly expressed in the limbic system, basal ganglia and hippocampus. These areas regulate emotion, motor activity and memory and cannabinoids play a central role in the neuromodulation of these functions. Disruptions of these systems lead to many CNS disorders and cannabinoids serve important functions in disease and health of the CNS. As modulators of intercellular chemical messaging, it is well established that major neurotransmitter nuclei and pathways are densely populated with the cannabinoid receptors. In addition to chemical messaging, cannabinoids have been proposed to modulate other neurological activities in the CNS including neuroprotection and neurogenesis.

Neuroprotection

Although the ancient Greeks were known to use cooling to treat head trauma and prevent greater injury, the concept of neuroprotection using hypothermia first entered the medical literature in 1940 (Jain, 2011). Fay in 1941 published an abstract in the journal *Anesthesiology* entitled "Observations on Prolonged Human Refrigeration" and reported on a woman with an ulcerating breast carcinoma treated with local refrigeration. By reducing the patient's body temperature to 90 °F, Fay found the breast area was much improved after five months of treatment with body cooling. The author's final comments in the abstract concluded with a positive comment that "One of the most gratifying results of generalized refrigeration is the relief of pain enjoyed by the patient after return to normal body temperatures" (Fay, 1941).

Although neurons can be damaged and die from multiple causes, neuroprotective mechanisms have shared features that limit the injury of the tissue. Trauma, stroke, oxidative stress, excitotoxicity, inflammation and mitochondrial dysfunction are all examples of conditions that injure the nervous system. In preclinical studies cannabinoids have been reported to protect the brain from these injuries by activating the CB_1 receptor (García-Arencibia *et al.*, 2007; Sagredo *et al.*, 2007). Of the two endocannabinoids, 2-AG has been found to mostly (but not exclusively) suppress oxidative stress and tumor necrosis factor alpha (TNF-α) (Gallily, Breuer and Mechoulam, 2000; Kreutz *et al.*, 2009) and is believed to be neuroprotective (Panikashvili *et al.*, 2001).

Using mice brain injury models, 2-AG was found to increase 10-fold within 4 hours after trauma and to remain elevated over 24 hours in the brain. After giving exogenous 2-AG to the injured mice (thus increasing the total 2-AG available to injured tissue), the percentage of water in brain tissue (edema) was reduced and neurological severity scores (NSS) improved with faster recovery of the animal (Panikashvili *et al.*, 2001).

Neuronal cell death is a common result of traumatic head injury and by addition of 2-AG neuroprotective effects were reported with reduction of infarction size by nearly 50%. When CB_1 antagonists were given with 2-AG following trauma, the neuroprotective effects were attenuated further demonstrating the protective role of CB_1 activation (Panikashvili et al., 2001).

In addition to CB_1, 2-AG also binds to CB_2 and this receptor could also be neuroprotective. As discussed earlier in Chapters 2 and 3, the CB_2 receptor has only a limited expression in the CNS and is more closely associated with immune cells in the periphery with only a small amount in microglial cells in the brain. In a recent report Magid et al. (2019) found the effects of two specific CB_2 agonists, α-pinene and camphor, to reduce brain injury using the rodent model of head injury measured by the NSS.

Although not a cannabinoid, both substances are terpenes and closely associated with the cannabis plant. α-Pinene is an aromatic terpene that gives off the scent of pine in marijuana and pine trees and is also present in dill and parsley. Camphor is a second aromatic terpene found within the wood in a species of evergreen trees in Asia. Although both α-pinene and camphor are strong CB_2 agonists, both bind very weakly to CB_1 (Magid et al., 2019).

Neuroprotection is an obvious important function for survival and multiple molecules other than 2-AG provide neuroprotection. Several "near-like" cannabinoids previously discussed in Chapter 3 have also been reported to have neuroprotective properties through binding to either the CB_1 or CB_2 receptors (Mechoulam et al., 2014).

Previously in Chapters 2 and 3 we also found that multiple molecules share enzymatic systems with endocannabinoids and can even be structurally similar to 2-AG or AEA. Arachidonoyl serine (ARA-S) is one such molecule and shares a molecular structure nearly identical to AEA differing only by one carboxy group. This difference is sufficient to prevent ARA-S from binding to either CB_1 or CB_2 receptors. In preclinical models of brain injury ARA-S has been found to be neuroprotective despite lack of affinity to the cannabinoid receptors (Zhang et al., 2010).

As the concept of neuroprotection becomes further understood, the therapeutic use of cannabinoids in trauma and neurodegenerative disease such as multiple sclerosis, ALS and Alzheimer's disease may come closer to reality.

Neurogenesis

Ramón y Cajal, frequently referred to as the "father of modern neuroscience," in 1913 wrote "Once development was ended, the fonts of growth and regeneration of the axons and dendrites dried up irrevocably. In adult centers, the nerve paths are something fixed and immutable: everything may die, nothing may be regenerated. It is for the science of the future to change, if possible, this harsh decree."(Colucci-D'Amato, Bonavita and di Porzio, 2006).

Neurogenesis is the birth of new neurons and from the nineteenth century and Cajal to recent times it was generally believed that birth of new neurons in the brain was terminated early in human development. In the 1970s tritiated thymidine became available to study the brain and studies revealed potential neurons in the hippocampus capable of neurogenesis (Hine and Das, 1974). Today it is recognized that under normal conditions in the adult brain the dentate gyrus (DG) in the hippocampus and the subventricular zone (SVC), an area adjacent to the thin ependymal layer that lines the lateral ventricles, are exceptions to this rule. When neurogenesis occurs in the DG, cells recently born differentiate into dentate granule cells, the predominate neuronal cell in the DG. In the SVC, activated cells migrate through the rostral migratory stream and differentiate into several types of olfactory neurons in the olfactory bulb. Neurogenesis may also occur within other areas of the brain including the neocortex and hypothalamus although this is less well accepted (Aimone, Deng and Gage, 2010).

Neural progenitor cells (PCs) are cells in the adult brain that have the potential to differentiate into other cells through neurogenesis. PCs are already more advanced than stem cells and differ from them in several important ways. One important difference is that PCs can differentiate only for a brief time into neurons before neurogenesis ceases. In addition, since many neurons that arose from activated PCs have limited life spans, neurogenesis may potentially be more important in the short-term plasticity of the brain rather than as a permanent replacement of lost cells (Campos et al., 2017).

In the DG and SVC the PCs are largely in a quiescent state and as undifferentiated cells share some similarities to astrocytes although the morphology and functionality is much different at maturation (Zhao, Deng and Gage, 2008). Niche-derived and intrinsic signals activate the process of neurogenesis and the PC differentiates through several closely regulated steps. Various neurotransmitters, growth factors and cytokines regulate this maturation and many activities in neurogenesis may be influenced by cannabinoids. Excitatory glutaminergic input into the dentate granular neurons and GABAergic inhibition may start the process of neurogenesis by activation of the quiescent PC. Other triggers including brain-derived neurotropic factor (BDNF), interleukin 6 (IL-6), TNFα and others also can initiate neurogenesis. External factors also can activate neurogenesis and include exercise, learning and antidepressant medications. As the activated PC differentiates into neuronal cells including neurons, astrocytes and oligodendrocytes, the cell matures and integrates itself into neural circuits. Activated PCs originating in the SVC, in contrast, as mentioned earlier, migrate towards the olfactory bulb and eventually differentiate into various granular olfactory neurons (Gage, 2000; Vadodaria and Gage, 2014).

Within the CNS, the ECS and especially the cannabinoid receptors are widely dispersed in the basal ganglia and limbic systems of the brain. The presence of the ECS within these structures underlies their critical role in the function and expression of emotion, memory and movement.

The limbic system is the emotional center of the brain and is where the feelings and memories important to human life dwell. This area was first described by Paul Broca in 1877 and the limbic system consists of several structures including the thalamus, hypothalamus, amygdala and hippocampus. The thalamus is an important relay station for sensory information to the brain and sensory input is directed to other areas of the brain including the cortex where our awareness of the external world is perceived.

Anxiety and Cannabinoids

Anxiety disorders are among the most common psychiatric conditions. Psychopharmacological treatments with benzodiazepines and antidepressants are commonly prescribed with some success but many patients remain symptomatic.

The growing social acceptance to use cannabis has unfortunately confused the treatment of anxiety since, for many patients, cannabis appears to have an anxiolytic effect while others report intense anxiety and even panic. These observations have left many unsure whether cannabinoids may become treatments in the long run or considered too dangerous for the anxious patient.

There is an extensive preclinical body of work but unfortunately only a few small human clinical trials evaluating the cannabinoids and anxiety. However, it is generally accepted that the effects of anxiety are modulated not only through the CB_1 receptor but also through other non-cannabinoid targets (Rubino, Zamberletti and Parolaro, 2015). From these studies it appears that activation of the CB_1 receptor by cannabinoids is anxiolytic although at higher doses anxiety symptoms can be induced. In addition, it is well known that environmental conditions including adverse stimuli play a part in inducing the expression of anxiety in both animal and human models (Viveros, Marco and File, 2005; Rey et al., 2012).

In one preclinical rodent study no differences were observed in inducing anxiety-like behaviors during normal conditions between genetically modified CB_1 knockout mice and normal wild-type mice. However, in an aversive condition environment, the CB_1 knockout mice exhibited behavioral changes consistent with anxiety (Jacob et al., 2009).

As we discussed earlier in Chapter 3, CB_1 receptors modulate both glutamate (excitatory) and GABAergic (inhibitory) neurons. In studies of rats genetically modified not to express glutamate receptors, CB_1 agonists have no effect on reducing anxiety. Similarly, in genetically modified rats without CB_1 receptors on GABAergic neurons, CB_1 agonists are ineffective as anxiolytics (Rey et al., 2012).

The absence or blockade of CB_1 receptors appears in general to increase anxiety and further supports the importance of the receptor in modulating anxiety. The effects of benzodiazepines that are effective anxiolytic drugs are blocked in mice without CB_1 receptors (Urigüen et al., 2004). Although most preclinical studies have demonstrated increased anxiety-like behaviors in the absence of CB_1 activation (Dubreucq et al., 2012), a few studies have reported no or reduced effects (Kathuria et al., 2003; Rubino et al., 2008). In addition, using pharmacological probes of CB_1 antagonists have also resulted in mixed outcomes in preclinical models of anxiety.

Although the general belief is that the anxiolytic effects of cannabinoids is mediated by CB_1 receptors, the CB_2 receptor may also play a role. Using CB_2 knockout mice, one investigator found increased responses to aversive stimuli similar to the results of other studies with CB_1 (Ortega-Alvaro et al., 2011). The significance of this finding is yet to be determined, however, since CB_2 expression in the CNS is extremely limited compared with that of CB_1.

Another approach in assessing the effects of endocannabinoids in anxiety is through inhibited degradation. Fatty acid amide hydrolase (FAAH) is a serine hydrolase that breaks down AEA and to a lesser extent 2-AG. Multiple preclinical studies using FAAH inhibitors also suggest that endocannabinoids have anxiolytic effects (Kathuria et al., 2003; O'Brien et al., 2013; Bluett et al., 2014). Further genetic models of mice without the gene for FAAH also were found to have less behaviors associated with anxiety. When FAAH is inhibited or mice genetically modified not to express the enzyme, increased synaptic availability of AEA and to a lesser degree 2-AG occurs. When treated with a CB_1 antagonist, this effect is lost demonstrating it is activation of the receptor by the cannabinoids that leads to the reduction of anxiety (Kathuria et al., 2003; Moreira et al., 2008; Rubino, Zamberletti and Parolaro, 2015).

Variation in FAAH expression in anxiolytic effects have also been reported in humans. In a pediatric study of over 1000 subjects between the ages of 3 and 21 years, Gee et al. (2016) reported that polymorphisms in FAAH altered AEA levels and the continued development of the frontal limbic circuitry. When these changes occurred by age 12 years, a reduction in the expression of anxiety-related behavior was observed. In the same report, the investigators studied genetically modified mice deficient in FAAH as an animal comparison. As the mice matured, similar reductions in anxiety-related behaviors were observed (Gee *et al.*, 2016).

The use of cannabis is also associated with precipitation of anxiety and panic. At first glance this seems confusing since activation of CB_1 receptors reduces anxiety. However, it is well accepted that there is a dose-dependent effect with higher concentrations of cannabinoids or greater potency of cannabis inducing anxiety. In Chapter 3 we discussed that cannabinoids also have significant binding affinities for non-cannabinoid receptors. At higher doses, AEA has been found to bind to the non-cannabinoid transient receptor potential vanilloid type 1 (TRPV1) receptor and this activation is believed to cause the anxiety-related behaviors observed in the animal models. This second receptor may explain the biphasic effects of cannabinoids that exhibit anxiolytic properties at low doses but induce anxiety at higher levels (Aguiar *et al.*, 2009). Further, blocking TRPV1 receptors in the prefrontal cortex (PFC) was found to reduce the rat anxiety-related behaviors (Aguiar *et al.*, 2009; Moreira *et al.*, 2012).

The role of 2-AG in the expression of anxiety is yet to be firmly established. However, in one study that inhibited 2-AG degradation by blocking its degradative enzyme monoacylglycerol lipase (MAGL), anxiety behaviors were blocked in an aversive environment (Bedse *et al.*, 2018). Additional studies will be required, however, before this question can be settled.

In addition to preclinical studies with endocannabinoids, there are several small and limited human trials using phytocannabinoids and observing the effect on anxiety. However, using the phytocannabinoid cannabidiol (CBD), these studies have generally supported the notion that anxiety symptoms may be relieved with CBD.

In one early study by Zuardi *et al.* (1993) the effects of CBD were reported in 40 healthy subjects in a comparison study with ipsapirone, an experimental drug known to be a partial agonist of $5HT_{1A}$. Subjects in this study were assigned to one of four conditions: CBD 300 mg PO, ipsapirone 5 mg PO TID, diazepam 10 mg PO daily or placebo. Subjects were asked to give a 4-minute presentation after having only 2 minutes of preparation time. They were then interrupted halfway through their presentation and their expression of anxiety measured. CBD was found to reduce post-stress anxiety similar to the other medication treatment groups (Zuardi *et al.*, 1993).

Crippa *et al.* (2003) in another early study evaluated normal volunteers without any personal or family history of anxiety. Subjects were given a larger dose of CBD at 400 mg PO or placebo in a randomized, crossover clinical trial. After dosing of the study drug, the subjects were assessed with the standard visual analog mood scale (VAMS) before and after dosage with CBD and underwent a single-photon emission computed tomography (SPECT). The study found a significant reduction in anxiety after CBD and an increased uptake of injected dye in the medial temporal cortex suggesting activity in the limbic and paralimbic areas of the brain (Crippa *et al.*, 2003). Although these early studies were limited to normal volunteers, later studies would evaluate patient populations.

Bergamaschi *et al.* (2011) studied 24 patients with social anxiety disorder (SAD) and 12 normal volunteers in a small, double-blind, placebo-controlled study. The patient group was divided into two groups of 12 each and treated with CBD 600 mg PO or placebo. Normal controls did not receive any medication in the study. After dosage with CBD or placebo, participants were given 2 minutes to prepare for a 4-minute oral presentation.

Once again, halfway through the presentation the subject was interrupted. Psychological measures including the VAMS and physiological measurements of skin conductance and arterial blood pressure were obtained both before the presentation and after the interruption.

The investigators found that CBD significantly reduced anxiety in the anticipation of the speech and after the interruption. The degree of cognitive impairment, physical discomfort and level of alertness were similar in patients that received CBD and normal controls without medication (Bergamaschi *et al.*, 2011).

Post-traumatic stress disorder (PTSD) is another frequent presentation of anxiety-like symptoms as a result of an external stimulus. Individuals that were physically close to the collapse of the World Trade Center (WTC) in 2001 were studied by Hill *et al.* (2013) and plasma endocannabinoids were collected from 46 subjects. These subjects were assessed initially by a structured psychiatric interview and 24 were diagnosed with PTSD and 22 as having no symptoms of PTSD. 2-AG, AEA and serum cortisol were measured in blood drawn from all subjects at 8:00 AM on the test day. A significant reduction of 2-AG was found in the PTSD patients but no difference in AEA or cortisol was found between groups. In PTSD patients with intrusive symptoms, a negative association with AEA was reported (Hill *et al.*, 2013).

Rimonabant was a CB_1 receptor antagonist approved for use in Europe in 2006. After only two years the product was withdrawn due to psychiatric adverse events and was never approved in the USA. Initially approved in Europe for weight loss with great anticipation, rimonabant was a CB_1 antagonist and possibly an inverse agonist as well. Although effective in suppressing appetite, the drug was also found to induce depression and suicidal ideation. In one study of over 800 patients in Europe, North America and Australia, 43.4% of patients treated with rimonabant reported treatment-emergent psychiatric adverse events (28.4% of placebo patients also reported adverse events in the study). Major depression, suicidal ideation and attempted suicide were the most severe events reported and at the same frequency as in placebo-treated patients. One patient on rimonabant successfully completed suicide (Nissen *et al.*, 2008).

Subsequent studies in normal volunteers without psychiatric history when given rimonabant also resulted in concerns about the psychiatric dangers associated with the blockade of the CB_1 receptor (Christensen *et al.*, 2007; Horder *et al.*, 2010). The significant adverse psychiatric events that occurred with CB_1 blockade with rimonabant was a remarkable observation and reinforces our understanding of the importance of the ECS and the CB_1 receptor in mood and anxiety disorders.

Even before rimonabant being withdrawn, there was already considerable preclinical evidence that indicated a reduction in ECS activity may be associated with depression. For example, genetically modified mice without CB_1 receptors had already demonstrated behaviors consistent with depression in several preclinical studies. It is believed that high stress (steroid secretion) inhibits neurogenesis. The ECS is neuroprotective of those areas that generate new tissue but steroids counter that effect. In addition, rodent models had found high corticosterone levels after stress which is consistent with overactivation of the hypothalamic–pituitary–adrenal (HPA) axis in severely depressed individuals (Urigüen *et al.*, 2004; Murphy, 2006).

There have also been a number of small clinical trials evaluating the ECS in depressed patients. Hill and Gorzalka (2009) reported a baseline reduction in circulating levels of AEA and 2-AG in blood of 15 medication-free depressed women compared with 15 normal controls. Samples for the "endocannabinoid-like" palmitoylethanolamide (PEA) and oleoy-lethanolamide were also collected. After obtaining the baseline samples, patients and controls were challenged using a social stressor test called Trier Social Stress Test (TSST). Following the stressor, serum 2-AG increased in the depressed women although AEA remained unchanged. Both PEA and OEA were reduced after the TSST challenge compared with their baseline (Hill and Gorzalka, 2009).

The experience of severe depression and suicidal ideation after CB_1 receptor antagonism by rimonabant and the reduction in circulating endocannabinoids in the bloodstream of women with major depression suggest hypofunction of the ECS in depressive disorders. Standard treatments for depression including antidepressants and electroconvulsive therapy have previously been reported to increase CB_1 expression in the limbic system (Gobbi et al., 2005; Gorzalka and Hill, 2011). Finally, sleep deprivation is another treatment for major depression and several preclinical studies have reported an increase in oleamide (OA) in cerebrospinal fluid (CSF) in sleep-deprived animals (Mendelson and Basile, 2001). Although OA is not an endocannabinoid it does bind to the cannabinoid receptor and is degraded by FAAH potentially influencing the availability of AEA.

The mood-elevating effects of marijuana have been known since the beginning of human use of cannabinoids. Activation of the CB_1 receptor by various agonists including THC can clearly lift mood and conversely, CB_1 antagonism can cause depression and suicidal ideation. Because of the absence of the psychoactive effects of other cannabinoids including CBD, these cannabinoids have been of great interest as a potential antidepressant medication. Recently a review of the medical literature evaluating CBD as an antidepressant treatment was published by Pinto et al. (2020). In this survey, the authors could not identify any well-conducted clinical trials that adequately evaluated the efficacy of CBD in treating mood disorders. Only two small case reports and four observational studies were found in the survey. No studies were identified that assessed depressed symptoms as the primary outcome. The authors concluded that there is lack of evidence that CBD has any effect in the treatment of mood disorders (Pinto et al., 2020).

Finally, several postmortem studies have evaluated the ECS in suicide victims with depression and have provided some limited insight into the role of cannabinoids in mood disorders. In one report by Hungund et al. (2004), brain tissue was examined from 10 individuals that had been diagnosed with major depression and died by suicide and was compared with brain tissue from a matched group of normal controls. They reported greater expression of the CB_1 receptor in the dorsal lateral PFC of the suicide group (Hungund et al., 2004).

Schizophrenia

In Chapter 5 we discussed the association between cannabis use and schizophrenia. It is now well accepted that cannabis use can increase the risk of developing schizophrenia earlier in life with greater severity of symptoms (Di Forti et al., 2019). Disturbances in the function of ECS have been reported not only after cannabis use but also in patients with schizophrenia (van Os et al., 2002; Hindley et al., 2020).

Leweke et al. (1999) first reported an increase in AEA and PEA in the CSF of 10 patients with schizophrenia when compared with matched controls, with similar findings later reported by Giuffrida et al., 2004. Subsequently, several small studies have collected markers of ECS activity from CSF, whole blood, plasma and serum. In a recent meta-analysis by Minichino *et al.* (2019) of this activity, 18 studies were identified that found increased levels of AEA of which 5 were measuring AEA levels in CSF and 9 in plasma or serum. Increased CB_1 expression was also found in peripheral immune cells of patients with schizophrenia compared with normal volunteers. The CB_2 receptor was also considered in the meta-analysis but there was insufficient data for the authors to comment on the function of this receptor in schizophrenia (Minichino *et al.*, 2019).

Other significant findings from this meta-analysis showed an association between the severity of positive and negative symptoms in schizophrenia and a decrease of AEA levels in CSF and increased expression of CB_1 receptors on peripheral immune cells. Poor cognition was also found to be associated with disruptions of the ECS with lower AEA in CSF and serum and reduced expression of ECS synthesizing enzymes. There was also a higher expression of ECS degrading enzymes and more abundant CB_1 and CB_2 receptors in the peripheral immune cells with decrements in cognitive functions (Minichino *et al.*, 2019).

The CB_1 and CB_2 receptors in schizophrenia have also been evaluated in other pre-clinical and clinical models. To date, the animal models have been inconsistent with increased CB_1 binding, no differences or even reduction in receptors reported (Zamberletti, Rubino and Parolaro, 2012; Rubino, Zamberletti and Parolaro, 2015).

Several postmortem studies of patients with schizophrenia have also reported unfortunately similar mixed findings. In human cortex, upregulation of the CB_1 receptor, no difference and reduction of the receptor have all been reported. Postmortem studies of schizophrenia can be complicated since reliable information on severity of illness, medication use and substance abuse is usually difficult to obtain. One report by Uriguen *et al.* (2009), however, found the density of CB_1 receptors was significantly reduced in patients treated with antipsychotics but higher in unmedicated schizophrenic patients.

In a more recent postmortem study of cortical tissue in 11 patients with schizophrenia and 11 matched controls without any psychiatric illness, the CB_1 and CB_2 receptors and the endocannabinoid degrading enzymes FAAH and MAGL were determined. Compared with the normal brains, the CB_1 mRNA in patient brains was decreased but was unrelated to prior medication history. No relationship was found between CB_2 receptor expression and the diagnosis of schizophrenia. However, the authors did acknowledge the small number of CB_2 receptors in the normal brain and the lack of highly selective CB_2 receptor agonists was a limitation of any findings about this receptor. In addition, no differences between patients and controls were found in the levels of the degrading enzymes FAAH and MAGL. The authors added there was no correlation between the PFC and the distribution of CB_1 mRNA, FAAH and MAGL in the brain. Controls, however, were found to have a positive correlation between these three ECS markers and the authors proposed an imbalance between the constituents of the ECS might occur in schizophrenia in contrast to the normal brain (Muguruza *et al.*, 2019).

In addition to the postmortem studies, several imaging studies are also available evaluating the ECS and schizophrenia. One in vivo PET imaging study of 67 patients with schizophrenia reported enhanced CB_1 binding in the cingulate and insular cortex. The cingulate cortex is related to the brain limbic system and the insular cortex is associated with the regulation of sensory input and emotional responses. Other areas of enhanced CB_1 binding were found in the nucleus accumbens, an area that is associated with reward and motivation, and in the pons (Ceccarini *et al.*, 2013).

Cannabidiol (CBD) and Schizophrenia

It is well established that THC can induce psychosis and that the ECS is altered in schizophrenia. This has led to inquiry whether the manipulation of endocannabinoids may provide options for treatment of schizophrenia.

CBD is a non-psychoactive phytocannabinoid that is known to mitigate many of the actions of THC. Zuardi *et al.* (1995) was the first to report using CBD in a case report of a 19-year-old female patient unable to tolerate antipsychotic medication. The patient was given CBD as monotherapy at dosages up to 1500 mg over four weeks. She responded with a decrease in the Brief Psychiatric Rating Scale (BPRS), a psychiatric scale that measures symptoms of psychosis and frequently used in clinical trials. Upon withdrawal, the author reported an exacerbation of her psychotic symptoms (Zuardi *et al.*, 1995).

In a more recent study, McGuire *et al.* (2018) reported an exploratory, eight-week, multi-center, double-blind, randomized, placebo-controlled study of 43 patients treated with CBD 1000 g/d as an adjunctive treatment to antipsychotic medication compared with 45 patients on antipsychotic medication and placebo. The author reported modest improvement in the positive symptoms of psychosis using objective rating scales and improvement in the blinded psychiatric clinical assessment. The strongest improvement was on motor speed and executive functioning with some enhancement also found in cognition (McGuire *et al.*, 2018).

Recently a systematic review of the medical literature on CBD and psychosis between 1970 and 2019 was published. Eight studies were identified in the survey by the authors to evaluate the outcome of CBD as a treatment for primary psychiatric disorders. A total of 210 patients were evaluated in this survey with four observational studies and four clinical trials identified. The authors concluded that the clinical data were mixed, and they could not conclude that CBD was effective as an antipsychotic or improved cognition. They did note that CBD appeared safe to use and was well tolerated compared with antipsychotic medication (Ghabrash *et al.*, 2020).

Bibliography

Aguiar, D. C. *et al.* (2009) 'Anxiolytic-like effects induced by blockade of transient receptor potential vanilloid type 1 (TRPV1) channels in the medial prefrontal cortex of rats', *Psychopharmacology*, 205(2), 217–225. doi:10.1007/s00213-009-1532-5.

Aimone, J. B., Deng, W. and Gage, F. H. (2010) 'Adult neurogenesis: integrating theories and separating functions', *Trends in Cognitive Sciences*, 14(7), pp. 325–337. doi:10.1016/j.tics.2010.04.003.

Bedse, G. *et al.* (2018) 'Therapeutic endocannabinoid augmentation for mood and anxiety disorders: comparative profiling of FAAH, MAGL and dual inhibitors', *Translational Psychiatry*, 8(1). doi:10.1038/s41398-018-0141-7.

Bergamaschi, M. M. *et al.* (2011) 'Cannabidiol reduces the anxiety induced by simulated public speaking in treatment-naïve social phobia patients', *Neuropsychopharmacology*, 36, 1219–1226. doi:10.1038/npp.2011.6.

Bluett, R. J. *et al.* (2014) 'Central anandamide deficiency predicts stress-induced anxiety: behavioral reversal through endocannabinoid augmentation', *Translational Psychiatry*, 4, e408. doi:10.1038/tp.2014.53.

Campos, A. C. *et al.* (2017) 'Plastic and neuroprotective mechanisms involved in the therapeutic effects of cannabidiol in psychiatric disorders, *Frontiers in Pharmacology*, 8, 269. doi:10.3389/fphar.2017.00269.

Ceccarini, J. *et al.* (2013) 'Increased ventral striatal CB1 receptor binding is related to negative symptoms in drug-free patients with schizophrenia', *NeuroImage*, 79, 304–312. doi:10.1016/j.neuroimage.2013.04.052.

Christensen, R. *et al.* (2007) 'Efficacy and safety of the weight-loss drug rimonabant: a meta-analysis of randomised trials', *The Lancet*, 370(9600), 1706–1713. doi:10.1016/S0140-6736(07)61721-8.

Colucci-D'Amato, L., Bonavita, V. and di Porzio, U. (2006) 'The end of the central dogma of neurobiology: stem cells and neurogenesis in adult CNS, *Neurological Sciences*, 27, 266–270. doi:10.1007/s10072-006-0682-z.

Crippa, J. A. *et al.* (2003) 'Effects of cannabidiol (CBD) on regional cerebral blood flow', *Neuropsychopharmacology*, 29(2), 417–426. doi:10.1038/sj.npp.1300340.

Di Forti, M. *et al.* (2019) 'High-potency cannabis and incident psychosis: correcting the causal assumption – authors' reply', *The Lancet Psychiatry*, 6(6), 466–467. doi:10.1016/S2215-0366(19)30176-2.

Dubreucq, S. *et al.* (2012) 'Genetic dissection of the role of cannabinoid type-1 receptors in the emotional consequences of repeated social stress in mice', *Neuropsychopharmacology*, 37(8), 1885–1900. doi:10.1038/npp.2012.36.

Fay, T. (1941) 'Observations on prolonged human refrigeration', *Anesthesiology*, 2(5), 347–348.

Gage, F. H. (2000) 'Mammalian neural stem cells', *Science*, 287(5457), 1433–1438. doi:10.1126/science.287.5457.1433.

Gallily, R., Breuer, A. and Mechoulam, R. (2000) '2-Arachidonylglycerol, an endogenous cannabinoid, inhibits tumor necrosis factor-α production in murine macrophages, and in mice', *European Journal of Pharmacology*, 406, R5–R7. doi:10.1016/s0014-2999(00)00653-1.

García-Arencibia, M. *et al.* (2007) 'Evaluation of the neuroprotective effect of cannabinoids in a rat model of Parkinson's disease: importance of antioxidant and cannabinoid receptor-independent properties', *Brain Research*, 1134(1), 162–170. doi:10.1016/j.brainres.2006.11.063.

Gee, D. G. *et al.* (2016) 'Individual differences in frontolimbic circuitry and anxiety emerge with adolescent changes in endocannabinoid signaling across species', *Proceedings of the National Academy of Sciences of the United States of America*, 113(16), 4500–4505. doi:10.1073/pnas.1600013113.

Ghabrash, M. F. *et al.* (2020) 'Cannabidiol for the treatment of psychosis among patients with schizophrenia and other primary psychotic disorders: a systematic review with a risk of bias assessment', *Psychiatry Research*, 286, 112890. doi:10.1016/j.psychres.2020.112890.

Giuffrida, A. *et al.* (2004) 'Cerebrospinal anandamide levels are elevated in acute schizophrenia and are inversely correlated with psychotic symptoms', *Neuropsychopharmacology*, 29(11), 2108–2114. doi:10.1038/sj.npp.1300558.

Gobbi, G. *et al.* (2005) 'Antidepressant-like activity and modulation of brain monoaminergic transmission by blockade of anandamide hydrolysis', *Proceedings of the National Academy of Sciences of the United States of America*, 102(51), 18620–18625. doi:10.1073/pnas.0509591102.

Gorzalka, B. B. and Hill, M. N. (2011) 'Putative role of endocannabinoid signaling in the etiology of depression and actions of antidepressants', *Progress in Neuro-Psychopharmacology and Biological Psychiatry*, 35(7), 1575–1585. doi:10.1016/j.pnpbp.2010.11.021.

Hill, M. N. *et al.* (2013) 'Reductions in circulating endocannabinoid levels in individuals with post-traumatic stress disorder following exposure to the world trade center attacks', *Psychoneuroendocrinology*, 38(12), 2952–2961. doi:10.1016/j.psyneuen.2013.08.004.

Hill, M. N. and Gorzalka, B. B. (2009) 'Impairments in endocannabinoid signaling and depressive illness', *JAMA: Journal of the American Medical Association*, 301(11), 1165–1166. doi:10.1001/jama.2009.369.

Hindley, G. *et al.* (2020) 'Psychiatric symptoms caused by cannabis constituents: a systematic review and meta-analysis', *The Lancet Psychiatry*, 7(4), 344–353. doi:10.1016/S2215-0366(20)30074-2.

Hine, R. and Das, G. D. (1974) 'Neuroembryogenesis in the hippocampal formation of the rat', *Zeitschrift für Anatomie und Entwicklungsgeschichte*, 144, 173–186. doi:10.1007/BF00519773.

Horder, J. *et al.* (2010) 'Reduced neural response to reward following 7 days treatment with the cannabinoid CB 1 antagonist rimonabant in healthy volunteers', *International Journal of Neuropsychopharmacology*, 13(8), 1103–1113. doi:10.1017/S1461145710000453.

Hungund, B. L. *et al.* (2004) 'Upregulation of CB1 receptors and agonist-stimulated [35S] GTPγS binding in the prefrontal cortex of depressed suicide victims', *Molecular Psychiatry*, 9(2), 184–190. doi:10.1038/sj.mp.4001376.

Jacob, W. *et al.* (2009) 'Endocannabinoids render exploratory behaviour largely independent of the test aversiveness: role of glutamatergic transmission', *Genes, Brain and Behavior*, 8(7), 685–698. doi:10.1111/j.1601-183X.2009.00512.x.

Jain, K. K. (2011) *The Handbook of Neuroprotection*. New York: Humana Press. doi:10.1007/978-1-61779-049-2.

Kathuria, S. *et al.* (2003) 'Modulation of anxiety through blockade of anandamide hydrolysis', *Nature Medicine*, 9(1), 76–81. doi:10.1038/nm803.

Klein, D. F. (2008) 'The loss of serendipity in psychopharmacology', *JAMA: Journal of the American Medical Association*, 299(9), 1063–1065. doi:10.1001/jama.299.9.1063.

Kreutz, S. *et al.* (2009) '2-Arachidonoylglycerol elicits neuroprotective effects on excitotoxically lesioned dentate gyrus granule cells via abnormal-cannabidiol-sensitive receptors on microglial cells', *Glia*, 57(3), 286–294. doi:10.1002/glia.20756.

Leweke, F. M. *et al.* (1999) 'Elevated endogenous cannabinoids in schizophrenia', *NeuroReport*, 10(8), 1665–1669. doi:10.1097/00001756-199906030-00008.

Magid, L. *et al.* (2019) 'Role of CB$_2$ receptor in the recovery of mice after traumatic brain injury', *Journal of Neurotrauma*, 36(11), 1836–1846. doi:10.1089/neu.2018.6063.

McGuire, P. *et al.* (2018) 'Cannabidiol (CBD) as an adjunctive therapy in schizophrenia: a multicenter randomized controlled trial', *American Journal of Psychiatry*, 175(3), 197–198. doi:10.1176/appi.ajp.2017.17030325.

Mechoulam, R. *et al.* (2014) 'Early phytocannabinoid chemistry to endocannabinoids and beyond', *Nature Reviews Neuroscience*, 15(11), 757–764. doi:10.1038/nrn3811.

Mendelson, W. B. and Basile, A. S. (2001) 'The hypnotic actions of the fatty acid amide, oleamide', *Neuropsychopharmacology*, 25(5), S36–S39. doi:10.1016/S0893-133X(01)00341-4.

Minichino, A. *et al.* (2019) 'Measuring disturbance of the endocannabinoid system in psychosis: a systematic review and meta-analysis', *JAMA Psychiatry*, 76(9), 914–923. doi:10.1001/jamapsychiatry.2019.0970.

Moreira, F. A. *et al.* (2008) 'Reduced anxiety-like behaviour induced by genetic and pharmacological inhibition of the endocannabinoid-degrading enzyme fatty acid amide hydrolase (FAAH) is mediated by CB1 receptors', *Neuropharmacology*, 54(1), 141–150. doi:10.1016/j.neuropharm.2007.07.005.

Moreira, F. A. *et al.* (2012) 'Cannabinoid type 1 receptors and transient receptor potential vanilloid type 1 channels in fear and anxiety-two sides of one coin?', *Neuroscience*, 204, 186–192. doi:10.1016/j.neuroscience.2011.08.046.

Muguruza, C. *et al.* (2019) 'Endocannabinoid system imbalance in the postmortem prefrontal cortex of subjects with schizophrenia', *Journal of Psychopharmacology*, 33(9), 1132–1140. doi:10.1177/0269881119857205.

Murphy, L. (2006) 'Endocannabinoids and endocrine function', in E. S. Onaivi, T. Sugiura and V. Di Marzo (eds.) *Endocannabinoids: The Brain and Body's Marijuana and Beyond*. Boca Raton: CRC Press. pp. 467–474.

Nissen, S. E. *et al.* (2008) 'Effect of rimonabant on progression of atherosclerosis in patients with abdominal obesity and coronary artery disease: The STRADIVARIUS randomized controlled trial', *JAMA: Journal of the American Medical Association*, 299(13), 1547–1560.

O'Brien, L. D. *et al.* (2013) 'Effect of chronic exposure to rimonabant and phytocannabinoids on anxiety-like behavior and saccharin palatability', *Pharmacology Biochemistry and Behavior*, 103(3), 597–602. doi:10.1016/j.pbb.2012.10.008.

Ortega-Alvaro, A. *et al.* (2011) 'Deletion of CB$_2$ cannabinoid receptor induces schizophrenia-related behaviors in mice', *Neuropsychopharmacology*, 36(7), 1489–1504. doi:10.1038/npp.2011.34.

Panikashvili, D. *et al.* (2001) 'An endogenous cannabinoid (2-AG) is neuroprotective after brain injury', *Nature*, 413(6855), 527–531. doi:10.1038/35097089.

Pinto, J. V. *et al.* (2020) 'Cannabidiol as a treatment for mood disorders: a systematic review', *Canadian Journal of Psychiatry*, 65 (4), 213–217. doi:10.1177/0706743719895195.

Rey, A. A. *et al.* (2012) 'Biphasic effects of cannabinoids in anxiety responses: CB1 and GABA$_B$ receptors in the balance of GABAergic and glutamatergic neurotransmission', *Neuropsychopharmacology*, 37(12), 2624–2634. doi:10.1038/npp.2012.123.

Rubino, T. *et al.* (2008) 'CB1 receptor stimulation in specific brain areas differently modulate anxiety-related behaviour', *Neuropharmacology*, 54(1), 151–160. doi:10.1016/j.neuropharm.2007.06.024.

Rubino, T., Zamberletti, E. and Parolaro, D. (2015) 'Endocannabinoids and mental disorders', in Pertwee, R. G. (ed.), *Endocannabinoids*. Springer International, pp. 261–283. doi:10.1007/978-3-319-20825-1_9.

Sagredo, O. *et al.* (2007) 'Cannabinoids and neuroprotection in basal ganglia disorders', *Molecular Neurobiology*, 36(1), 82–91. doi:10.1007/s12035-007-0004-3.

Urigüen, L. *et al.* (2004) 'Impaired action of anxiolytic drugs in mice deficient in cannabinoid CB$_1$ receptors', *Neuropharmacology*, 46(7), 966–973. doi:10.1016/j.neuropharm.2004.01.003.

Urigüen, L. *et al.* (2009) 'Immunodensity and mRNA expression of A$_{2A}$ adenosine, D$_2$ dopamine, and CB$_1$ cannabinoid receptors in postmortem frontal cortex of subjects with schizophrenia: effect of antipsychotic treatment', *Psychopharmacology*, 206(2), 313–324. doi:10.1007/s00213-009-1608-2.

Vadodaria, K. C. and Gage, F. H. (2014) 'SnapShot: adult hippocampal neurogenesis', *Cell*, 156(5), 1114–1114.e1. doi:10.1016/j.cell.2014.02.029.

van Os, J. *et al.* (2002) 'Cannabis use and psychosis: a longitudinal population-based study', *American Journal of Epidemiology*, 156(4), 319–327. doi:10.1093/aje/kwf043.

Viveros, M. P., Marco, E. M. and File, S. E. (2005) 'Endocannabinoid system and stress and anxiety responses', *Pharmacology Biochemistry and Behavior*, 81(2), 331–342. doi:10.1016/j.pbb.2005.01.029.

Zamberletti, E., Rubino, T. and Parolaro, D. (2012) 'The endocannabinoid system and schizophrenia: integration of evidence', *Current Pharmaceutical Design*, 18(32), 4980–4990. doi:10.2174/138161212802884744.

Zhang, X. *et al.* (2010) 'Endocannabinoid-like N-arachidonoyl serine is a novel pro-angiogenic mediator', *British Journal of Pharmacology*, 160(7), 1583–1594. doi:10.1111/j.1476-5381.2010.00841.x.

Zhao, C., Deng, W. and Gage, F. H. (2008) 'Mechanisms and functional implications of adult neurogenesis', *Cell*, 132(4), 645–660. doi:10.1016/j.cell.2008.01.033.

Zuardi, A. W. *et al.* (1993) 'Effects of ipsapirone and cannabidiol on human experimental anxiety', *Journal of Psychopharmacology*, 7 (1_suppl), 82–88. doi:10.1177/026988119300700112.

Zuardi, A. W. *et al.* (1995) 'Antipsychotic effect of cannabidiol', *Journal of Clinical Psychiatry*, 56(10), 485–486.

Cannabinoids in Sleep and Circadian Rhythms

The death of each day's life, sore labour's bath, balm of hurt minds, great natures' second course, chief nourisher in life's feast.

William Shakespeare, Macbeth

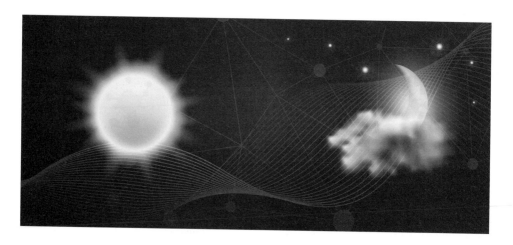

- Although there are no cannabinoid-based medicines approved for use in sleep disorders, the Institute of Medicine in 2017 concluded that there was moderate evidence that cannabinoids, especially nabiximols, were effective for short-term sleep disturbances.
- The endocannabinoid system is highly expressed in brain nuclei and pathways associated with sleep.
- Both 2-arachidonoylglycerol (2-AG) and N-arachidonoylethanolamide (anandamide; AEA) modulate the activities of neurotransmitters associated with sleep including gamma-aminobutyric acid (GABA) and glutamate.
- Preclinical studies of rapid eye movement sleep (REM sleep) deprivation suggest that cannabinoid 1 (CB$_1$) receptor expression and activity increase during REM sleep.
- In a small human study 2-AG exhibited a circadian rhythm with the lowest point at 4 AM.
- The chemically synthesized Δ^9-tetrahydrocannabinol (THC) dronabinol has been found to reduce apneic events in human studies of obstructive sleep apnea (OSA).

Disturbances in sleep are frequent complaints and numerous remedies have been proposed since the beginning of recorded time. Probably cannabis use has existed for just as long for many things including sleep and is still used many nights for a way of having a good sleep.

The continued interest in cannabis and cannabinoids potentially holds great promise in the treatment of sleep disorders. In this chapter we will review selected preclinical and clinical studies to provide the clinician (and their patients) information about sleep and cannabinoids and about the potential for future development of cannabinoids to treat sleep disorders. Already there are numerous personal testimonies, anecdotal reports and promotional claims that cannabinoids are helpful remedies for sleep complaints. However, the clinician should be aware that no regulatory agency in any country has approved cannabinoid products to treat sleep disorders.

A growing number of countries and multiple states in the USA have legalized marijuana for medical use although this is not the same as a regulatory approval to prescribe a drug for clinical use. A drug must be shown in adequately powered, randomized clinical trials to demonstrate both safety and efficacy in the treatment of a specific disease. In addition, once approved the drug is monitored for continuing safety and efficacy and can be withdrawn from the market. Although medical marijuana is now widely available and highly promoted, adequate efficacy and safety data remain to be collected.

In Chapter 5 we briefly discussed the many concerns regarding the safety of cannabinoids. These concerns still remain despite the intense promotional and social pressures to use cannabinoids for therapeutic or recreational purposes. Although the emerging data are promising and deserve further study, clinicians should always prioritize the safety of their patient before making any recommendation to use a drug where information is incomplete, including any of the cannabinoids.

Several professional medical societies have cautioned against the use of cannabinoids in the care of patients. In 2017 the National Academy of Medicine convened a committee of expert scientists and clinicians and published *The Health Effects of Cannabis and Cannabinoids: The Current State of Evidence and Recommendations for Research* (National Academy of Sciences, Engineering, and Medicine, 2017). This was an update from an earlier report in 1999 and reviewed the medical literature published in the intervening years. Over 24,000 articles were identified and data from over 10,000 were included in the report (Piomelli *et al.*, 2017).

This report concluded that there was only moderate evidence that cannabinoids, primarily nabiximols, are an effective treatment to improve short-term outcomes in individuals with sleep disturbance associated with obstructive sleep apnea (OSA) syndrome and several related medical conditions including fibromyalgia, chronic pain and multiple sclerosis (National Academy of Sciences, Engineering, and Medicine, 2017).

An Introduction to Sleep

The sleep-promoting properties of cannabis have been recognized for centuries stretching back to the ancient Chinese and Ayurvedic culture of India. In the eighteenth century, the great botanist Carolus Linnaeus also recognized these effects of cannabis on sleep and classified cannabis initially as a narcotic.

Until 1917, little was known about the physical basis of sleep. During the pandemic of 1917 now referred to as the "Spanish flu," Constantin von Economo presented to the Vienna

Psychiatric Society seven patient cases that had presented with excessive somnolence and paralysis. von Economo termed the illness "encephalitis lethargica" because of the profound sleep that sometimes led to coma and related motor symptoms suggestive of Parkinson's disease. Although the pandemic was known as a highly infectious respiratory illness that spread throughout Europe and North America eventually infecting over 500 million people, many patients also had degrees of somnolence and motor impairment. Although the viral etiology was unknown to von Economo, after examining the autopsied brains from patients with encephalitis lethargica, he realized that the Spanish flu also had effects on the central nervous system (CNS). From the postmortem studies of patients that had died from the pandemic, he found damage from this infection localized in the posterior hypothalamus and rostral midbrain in the brain causing profound drowsiness and coma. In contrast, injury to the anterior hypothalamus and basal forebrain would result in insomnia. von Economo's insight that the sleep–wake cycle was associated with specific brain structures and not a function of the whole brain provided the beginning of our understanding of sleep today.

Other advances added to our knowledge of sleep during the same period of the twentieth century. In 1924, Hans Berger, a German psychiatrist intrigued about the possibility of telepathy and brain function, recorded the electrical activity of the human brain for the first time. This procedure, termed the electroencephalogram (EEG), consisted of electrodes applied to the scalp that recorded the underlying brain electrical activity. Berger observed when the eyes were closed brain electrical activities occurred between 7 and 13 times per second. These waves were named "alpha waves" and were suppressed by faster "beta" waves when the eyes were opened. Berger's discoveries were originally met with skepticism and only after later replication by others was the importance of Berger's observations recognized.

Other advances in describing the electrical activity of the brain and sleep were soon to follow. Alfred Loomis was an entrepreneur interested in electricity and radio and radar transmissions. In 1937 he discovered large, peaked waves on the EEG of sleeping humans, later termed K-complex waves. These high-voltage waves were quickly followed during the EEG recording by bursts of low-voltage waves that were named sleep spindles. The discovery of the K-complex and associated sleep spindles led to the understanding that sleep was not a single state but is divided into several stages that differ in electrical activity and physiological function. By the 1950s, Nathaniel Kleitman and his students Eugene Aserinsky and William Dement described a stage of sleep characterized by a mixed frequency EEG that was reminiscent of the waking EEG but was associated with hypotonia and rapid excursions of the eyes (Dement and Kleitman, 1957). This stage of sleep was named rapid eye movement sleep (REM sleep) and was later established to be physiologically very distinct from non-REM sleep. Eventually other physiological data including heart rate and respiration were collected in addition to the sleep stages and the procedure now known as polysomnography (PSG) was established. Today, the PSG has become the tool of the clinical sleep laboratory to diagnose and treat numerous sleep complaints including sleep apnea, narcolepsy and periodic leg movements in sleep. Later in this chapter we will discuss how the PSG was used to study the effects of phytocannabinoids and synthetic cannabinoids on sleep.

The Waking Brain

Although the brain stem was originally believed to be the source of wakefulness, later other centers within the brain were identified that were associated with wakefulness. As these brain centers and pathways that enabled communication between cells were identified, the complexity of the sleep–wake cycle began to emerge.

Multiple types of neurotransmitters that are modulated by cannabinoids are involved in the initiation, maintenance and termination of the sleep–wake cycle. Neurons containing acetylcholine (cholinergic) serve a prominent role in wakefulness. Cholinergic projections from the brain stem laterodorsal (LDT) and pedunculopontine (PPT) tegmental nuclei terminate on centers in the thalamus where sensory information is then relayed to higher cortical centers through the thalamocortical pathways. Another cholinergic pathway from the brain stem to the cortex and basal forebrain bypasses the thalamic relay circuit and originates in the reticular formation in the midbrain and pons. A second family of neurotransmitters are the monoamines and these pathways project directly into the cortex and serve a prominent role in wake and alertness. Norepinephrine, originating from the pontine locus coeruleus, serotonin, from the dorsal raphe neurons, and histamine, from the tubular mammillary neurons, together serve as an ensemble of chemical signaling to the cortex. Other wake-inducing neurons are found in the lateral hypothalamus and have recently been identified to contain orexin (also called hypocretin). These neurons are most active during wakefulness and times requiring high alertness. Projections from the orexin-containing hypothalamic nuclei connect to other wake-promoting centers including the raphe nuclei and basal forebrain. With inactivity of the orexin system irresistible sleep and cataplexy occurs and is associated with the sleep disorder narcolepsy. The endocannabinoid system (ECS) (especially cannabinoid 1 [CB_1] receptors) is especially abundant throughout the brain structures and circuits that underlie wakefulness.

The Sleeping Brain

Once it was recognized that the electrical patterns recorded by the EEG changed during sleep, the observed distinctive patterns were classified as sleep stages. Non-REM sleep is divided into four stages of sleep with stages three and four referred to as slow wave sleep. REM sleep is a separate and unique stage of sleep not included in non-REM sleep.

Various functions are served by non-REM sleep. Loss of autonomic function with a slowing of heart rate and drop in blood pressure and cardiac output may occur (Burdick et al., 1970; Coccagna et al., 1971) and within the first hour or two of non-REM sleep, a surge of growth hormone is released into the bloodstream (Mendelson et al., 1979). In addition to activities, consolidation of declarative memory occurs during non-REM sleep and differs from memory consolidation processes in REM sleep (Tucker et al., 2006; Stickgold, 2013).

Gamma-aminobutyric acid (GABA) is an amino acid transmitter associated with non-REM sleep. GABA is the most abundant inhibitory neurotransmitter in the brain and closely influenced by the ECS. It is present in high concentrations within the brain and spinal cord but is found only in trace amounts in other tissues of the body including the peripheral nervous system. Compared with other neurotransmitter systems such as the monoamines, GABA is highly concentrated within the CNS and located in discreet nuclei within the brain. Approximately 30% of CNS synapses are believed to be GABA and strongly influenced by the endocannabinoid system (ECS).

GABA serves as the major inhibitory neurotransmitter on chemical messaging and is frequently associated with sleep disorders and neuropsychiatric disease. Epilepsy, schizophrenia, mood disorders and neurodegenerative disorders have all been associated with disturbances in GABA function in addition to sleep disorders. Cannabinoids modulate many neurotransmitter systems and the interaction between GABA neurons and cannabinoids is well established.

When von Economo observed lesions within the anterior hypothalamus and basal forebrain in the postmortem brain of patients with encephalitis lethargica, he postulated the existence of a sleep center in the anterior hypothalamus. Over 80 years later, the proposed sleep center was identified in the ventrolateral preoptic nucleus (VLPO), an area within the anterior hypothalamus that is especially active during sleep and rich in GABA-containing neurons (Sherin *et al.*, 1996). Within the VLPO, GABA plays an important role in sleep by inhibition of ascending pathways from the brain stem and the orexin system. The interaction between the VLPO and the arousal/orexin systems has been proposed by some to serve as an on–off switch for the sleep–wake cycle.

Positioned lateral to the suprachiasmatic nucleus (SCN), the master circadian clock in the body, the VLPO surprisingly has little direct connection to the clock (Chou *et al.*, 2003). Apparently, communication from the SCN (the body's internal clock) to the VLPO (the on–off switch of sleep) proceeds through a relay communication in the dorsomedial nucleus. Through this indirect route, critical information regarding the external environment (day–night; seasonal) is communicated to the VLPO that controls the internal sleep–wake cycle. Lesions of the dorsomedial nucleus have been reported to disrupt or even terminate the normal regulation of the circadian organization of sleep (Lu *et al.*, 2000).

REM Sleep and the Brain

As noted earlier, REM sleep was first described in the early 1950s using the sleep EEG. This discovery was shortly followed with the observation that dreaming was associated with REM sleep (Dement and Kleitman, 1957). Michel Jouvet reported in 1959 the persistence of REM sleep in cats that were decorticated. This established the role of the brain stem in the generation of REM sleep. When projections from the brain stem were severed from higher centers in the brain, the decorticated cat appeared to "act out" dreams without the influence of the controlling regions of the brain (Jouvet and Michel, 1959).

The pons and brain stem reticular formation are now accepted as the origin of REM sleep. Cholinergic neurons in the LDT and PPT nuclei are most active during REM sleep and terminate upon glutamate-containing neurons in the sublaterodorsal tegmental nucleus (SLD). Within the SLD, these activated neurons communicate to inhibitory interneurons and turn off motor activity to produce atonia in REM sleep (Lu, Sherman and Saper, 2006).

Other neurons in the brain stem reticular formation terminate rostral in the lateral geniculate nucleus in the thalamus (Nishino, 2013). From the thalamus, pathways then project to the visual occipital cortex. This circuit generates activity referred to as the ponto-geniculo-occipital (PGO) waves, originates in the pons and becomes most active just before REM sleep (Brooks and Bizzi, 1963). PGO waves have been identified in multiple animal species and reinforced the importance of the pons in the origination of REM sleep.

Finally, REM sleep is remarkable not only for the central role of the cholinergic system, but for the virtual absence of the monoamine systems that are involved in wakefulness. Norepinephrine, serotonin and histamine, chemical messengers that communicate during wake, are virtually silent during REM sleep. This reciprocal interaction between the cholinergic and monoamine system has led to several models of a REM on/REM off model of control (McCarley, 2011). The ECS has a prominent presence in both the monoamine and cholinergic circuits.

Endocannabinoids and Sleep

Endocannabinoids are bioactive lipids produced in cellular lipid membranes that bind to the CB_1 and CB_2 receptors and several families of non-cannabinoid receptors. In the early 1990s N-arachidonoylethanolamide (anandamide; AEA) and 2-arachidonoylglycerol (2-AG), two lipid molecules derived from arachidonic acid, were identified as endocannabinoids. Later, other lipid molecules were discovered that bind to the cannabinoid receptors and other non-cannabinoid receptors. These additional receptors included transient receptor potential vanilloid type 1 receptor (TRPV1), G protein receptor 55 (GPR55) and peroxisome proliferator-activated receptor-alpha (PPARα).

Oleamide, virodhamine and 2-arachidonyl glyceryl ether (2-AGE) are examples of these "endocannabinoid-like" molecules. Although they are not classified as endocannabinoids, they do demonstrate many of the properties of AEA and 2-AG in sleep and bind to the cannabinoid receptor.

N-acylethanolamides (NAEs) are another class of related lipid molecules and include oleoylethanolamide (OEA) and palmitoylethanolamide (PEA). NAEs are synthesized and degraded through pathways shared with AEA and 2-AG but do not bind to cannabinoid receptors. In part because of the shared enzymatic metabolic processes, NAEs may compete with endocannabinoids for access to synthesis and degradation. This competition may indirectly influence the availability of the endocannabinoids and their effect on sleep.

The ECS and Sleep and the Circadian Clock

The sleep–wake cycle is now known to be a complex communication between brain nuclei and the brain stem, diencephalon and cortex. The coordination of the sleep–wake cycle is overseen by a circadian clock located in the SCN found above the optic chiasm. Communication within this network is provided by several neurotransmitters including the inhibitory amino acid GABA, monoamines including norepinephrine, dopamine and histamine, acetylcholine and orexin. Closely associated with these networks is the ECS modulating these chemicals in their conversation.

Circadian Rhythms and the Endocannabinoid System

The term circadian means "about one day." Circadian rhythms are biological cycles of approximately 24 hours in duration regulated by the SCN located in the hypothalamus. The SCN controls the timing of sleep and the coordination of circadian rhythms in the body such as core body temperature, cortisol secretion and intraocular pressure (Aschoff, 1973). The SCN receives input about the environmental photoperiod through the retinohypothalamic tract and synchronizes internal circadian rhythms to the geophysical world (Moore and Lenn, 1972).

Preclinical animal studies have found that cannabinoids do not influence the sensory input of light cues from the environment but are more likely to modify the adjustment (termed entrainment) of the SCN to the external light–dark cycle. GABA appears to be an important neurotransmitter in cellular communications within the SCN (Liu and Reppert, 2000; Shirakawa *et al.*, 2000) and cannabinoids are known to inhibit GABA neurons through presynaptic binding to the CB_1 receptor. CB_1 receptors have also been found to be highly expressed in the hypothalamus and the SCN (Sanford, Castillo and Gannon, 2008; Sládek, Houdek and Sumová, 2019).

Core body temperature is a circadian rhythm closely associated with the sleep–wake cycle and controlled by the SCN. In a rat study of chronic one-week administration of low- or high-dose Δ^9-tetrahydrocannabinol (THC) compared with no treatment, the circadian rhythm of core body temperature after THC was inverted compared with no treatment. After discontinuation of THC, a 12-hour change in peak temperature was reported (Perron, Tyson and Sutherland, 2001).

In Chapter 3 we discussed the ECS and noted it consists of the endocannabinoids AEA and 2-AG, synthesis and degradation of AEA and 2-AG through separate enzymatic pathways, and at least two cannabinoid (CB_1 and CB_2) receptors. The CB_1 receptor density in the brain has been found in preclinical studies to vary during the day while CB_2 receptor density apparently remains constant (Martínez-Vargas et al., 2003; Rueda-Orozco et al., 2010). In a study of rat brain (a nocturnal species), the CB_1 receptor density varied between the dark active phase and the light inactive phase with the highest receptor density in the inactive phase.

In addition to the circadian changes reported with the CB_1 receptor, the endocannabinoids AEA and 2-AG also are expressed with a circadian rhythm in large areas of the rat brain including hypothalamus, hippocampus, nucleus accumbens, prefrontal cortex, striatum and pontine brain stem (Valenti et al., 2004; Murillo-Rodriguez, Désarnaud and Prospéro-García, 2006) with AEA peaking during the active dark phase of the rat. AEA in rat cerebrospinal fluid (CSF) was also found to peak during the light inactive phase (Murillo-Rodriguez, Désarnaud and Prospéro-García, 2006). Since endocannabinoids are produced on demand and are not stored in cell vesicles, further studies are required to understand the regulation of these reported circadian patterns. The serine hydrolase enzymes involved in the synthetic and catalytic pathways of endocannabinoids have also been found to be expressed in a diurnal pattern. It is likely that the circadian variation in AEA and 2-AG are markers for the circadian enzymatic activity of fatty acid amide hydrolase and monoacylglycerol lipase pathways.

Human data have also shown an association between expression of the ECS and the circadian system. Blood samples of 2-AG and 2-oleoylglycerol (2-OG), an NAE that is a structural analog of 2-AG, were obtained from 14 normal subjects starting in the late evening and continuing for 24 hours at hourly intervals. The lowest point for plasma 2-AG was found at 4 AM. 2-AG levels then gradually increased during the day before peaking during the early afternoon. 2-OG was drawn at the same time as 2-AG. Although the circadian rhythm of 2-OG was similar to 2-AG, the peak was less dramatic and had a limited duration. As both 2-OG and 2-AG are synthesized and degraded by the same enzymes, the similar results suggest a shared circadian regulation of the two lipid molecules (Hanlon et al., 2015).

Recently the human circadian profile in blood of AEA has been reported. In this study, Bowles et al. (2019) obtained blood samples from 13 healthy volunteers and reported a diurnal variation in AEA in non-lean individuals. A circadian rhythm of AEA was reported in non-lean volunteers. AEA in lean individuals, in contrast, appeared relatively constant with no rhythm found (Bowles et al., 2019). The authors hypothesized that body mass may influence the circadian levels of circulating endocannabinoids.

In 1994, a long chain, unsaturated lipid similar to sphingosine was isolated from the CSF of sleep-deprived cats (Lerner et al., 1994). The molecule initially was named cerebrodiene. The following year after further study the molecule was identified as oleamide and found to induce sleep in preclinical animal models (Cravatt et al., 1995; Mendelson and Basile, 2001) and in humans (Nichols et al., 2007). Additional studies using sleep EEG found that administration of oleamide produced non-REM sleep (Basile, Hanus and Mendelson, 1999). When a synthetic CB_1 antagonist was given in the preclinical model, the previous increase in non-REM sleep by oleamide was blocked suggesting that sleep induction was mediated through the CB_1 receptor (Mendelson and Basile, 1999).

Only a few studies of AEA on sleep are available and the results have been inconsistent. In a 2009 report of 20 human normal subjects, CSF and plasma levels of AEA and the structural analog OEA were collected over 24 hours after sleep deprivation. AEA levels in CSF were unchanged compared with the baseline state but OEA showed a significant increase from baseline (Koethe et al., 2009). Although OEA does not bind to the cannabinoid receptor, it does have significant affinity for PPARα and TRPV1. OEA is well known for its activities in feeding, body weight and lipid metabolism probably through binding to the PPARα receptor. The authors speculated that OEA serves as an anti-inflammatory and protects the brain from the oxidative stimulant effects of sleep deprivation.

In 2010 in another human study of five normal volunteers, AEA plasma levels were collected in two phases: before the first night of sleep, the following morning after awakening, and then in the early evening prior to the second sleep period (Vaughn et al., 2010). AEA levels after a night of sleep were highest in the morning suggesting AEA increases during the sleep period. In the second phase of the study, subjects underwent 24 hours of sleep deprivation. Plasma levels of AEA again rose during the night in spite of forced sleep deprivation. During the following day awake, three of the five subjects showed a continued rise in plasma AEA in contrast to the first phase when they were allowed to sleep at night. Since the first phase of the study showed a decrease in plasma AEA in all five subjects in the early evening, the authors suggested that sleep deprivation results in dysregulation of AEA in plasma.

Endocannabinoids may also play a role in the generation of REM sleep. REM sleep deprivation is known to result in a robust rebound effect in REM sleep when the restrictions on sleep are removed. In a study in rats of REM sleep deprivation followed by a 2-hour sleep rebound period, an increase in the number of CB_1 receptors was found with a decrease in mRNA in the brain stem (Martinez-Vargas et al., 2003). The authors of the study postulated that the CB_1 receptor expression and activity increase during REM sleep. In a separate rat study of REM sleep deprivation and rebound, a CB_1 antagonist blocked the expected increase in REM sleep after deprivation (Navarro et al., 2003).

As noted earlier in this chapter, the cholinergic system plays a major role in REM sleep while monoamine activity is quiescent. In the pontine tegmentum, the previously described cholinergic PPT and LDT nuclei neurons play a critical role in the initiation and regulation of REM sleep. Injection of AEA into the PPT nuclei resulted in an increase in non-REM and REM sleep. When a CB_1 receptor antagonist was added to the endocannabinoid, the increase in non-REM and REM sleep was blocked, demonstrating the importance of the CB_1 receptor in initiation of non-REM and REM sleep (Murillo-Rodríguez et al., 2001).

Information on 2-AG and REM sleep is limited. When 2-AG was infused into the lateral hypothalamus, sleep was increased. With the addition of a CB_1 receptor blocker, the increase in sleep was reversed (Martinez-Vargas et al., 2013). This result suggests that activation of the CB1 receptor in the lateral hypothalamus activates non-cholinergic mechanisms that initiate REM sleep.

Cannabis and Sleep

As discussed in Chapters 1 and 2, *Cannabis sativa* contains more than 100 different phytocannabinoids, terpenes and flavonoids. In addition, environmental factors including length of sunshine, temperature and moisture play significant roles in the overall composition of the plant and cultivation of cultivars of higher THC and lower cannabidiol (CBD) potency results in different effects from smoked cannabis. As a result, there is great variability in cannabis and the initial studies on sleep are frequently difficult to interpret because of the inconsistency of the composition of the smoked plant.

Earlier in this chapter we briefly presented some of the complexities associated with sleep. The environment where sleep is desired and various psychological factors obviously influence sleep and subjective differences in the motivation to use cannabis either for its psychoactive effects or for sedation can influence the outcome of the study. For example, many habitual users of cannabis describe their sleep as improved and satisfactory (Schofield et al., 2006; Reinarman et al., 2011). Real-world observational studies, however, indicate an increased risk of sleep disorders among cannabis users (Wong, Brower and Zucker, 2009). Further, withdrawal from habitual use of cannabis frequently is associated with sleep disruption and reduction of quality of sleep even when no preexisting sleep complaint was present.

The sleep EEG and the PSG were first applied to study the effects of cannabis in the 1970s. These early studies used the objective measurements of the sleep laboratory to describe the effects of cannabis in physically healthy insomniacs and found a decrease time to sleep onset and reduction in time asleep (Cousens and DiMascio, 1973). Changes in sleep architecture also were reported by Pivik et al. (1972) in healthy normal volunteers with an increase in slow wave sleep and reduction in latency to sleep onset. These first reports were consistent with the long-held belief that cannabis use resulted in falling asleep faster and increasing deeper sleep. Subsequent studies followed with habitual cannabis users at high doses of THC found to have increases in slow wave sleep (Barratt, Beaver and White, 1974) or a reduction in REM sleep and rebound of REM sleep upon withdrawal (Feinberg et al., 1975, 1976). Surprisingly, although these studies continued to confirm changes in sleep architecture as a result of cannabis use, these studies of habitual users did not replicate the earlier findings of falling asleep faster and sleeping longer.

More recently, understanding the effects of individual cannabinoids and dosages has started to be investigated. As discussed in Chapter 2, THC and CBD are two of the most common cannabinoids present in cannabis and have received the most interest as single agents used in sleep disorders.

THC administered at 15 mg before sleep to healthy volunteers in the sleep laboratory did not result in any change in sleep. However, the next morning subjects reported hangover effects of drowsiness with reduced cognition (Nicholson et al., 2004). When CBD 15 mg was combined with THC 15 mg no significant change in overnight sleep was recorded but subjects appeared less hungover the next day. This suggests that CBD at 15 mg is activating and can reverse the residual daytime effects of THC.

CBD may have dose-related effects on sleep. At higher doses, CBD appears to have sedating properties as demonstrated by preclinical rodent sleep EEG studies (Murillo-Rodríguez et al., 2006). There is limited data on higher doses of CBD in man but one report of over 2000 patient self-reports treated with nabiximols, discussed in Chapter 4 (a roughly 1:1 combination of THC and CBD), found that patients in clinical trials treated with CBD for various disease including multiple sclerosis, peripheral neuropathic pain, intractable cancer pain and rheumatoid arthritis were found to have subjectively good or very good sleep quality.

Cannabinoids may also be important in OSA (Babson, Sottile and Morabito, 2017). Sleep apnea is a disorder of breathing during sleep that results in obstruction of breathing during sleep and impairment the following day. Frequently associated with increased body weight, an estimated 11.9% of middle-aged men are estimated to have OSA (Newman et al., 2005). Animal studies that used rats with sleep apneic events during sleep found that both THC and the endocannabinoid-like oleamide reduced apneic events indicating that CB_1 receptor agonist activity may diminish apneic events (Carley et al., 2002). More recent investigations in the rat model used dronabinol, a synthetic THC reviewed in Chapter 4, in two rat studies and also found reduction in apneic events (Calik, Radulovacki and Carley, 2014). Proof-of-concept human studies of dronabinol have now been conducted with demonstration by PSG of reduced apneas and improved sleep (Prasad, 2013; Carley et al., 2018).

Discontinuation of cannabis from habitual users has been reported to disrupt sleep. These disruptions are characterized by changes in sleep patterns, vivid dreams, aggression and anxiety among other complaints associated with stopping cannabis use (Budney et al., 2003). Although some have claimed only limited dependence to cannabis occurs, more recent studies of cannabis confirm the presence of impaired sleep similar to the complaints and time course encountered in nicotine withdrawal. Using sleep laboratory to assess withdrawal from cannabis in heavy users, a delay in falling asleep, decrease in the time asleep with multiple awakenings, increased periodic leg movements and a reduction in percent of REM sleep have been reported (Bolla et al., 2010).

Bibliography

Aschoff, J. (1973) 'Circadian rhythms: influences of internal and external factors on the period measured in constant conditions', Zeitschrift für Tierpsychologie, 49(3), 225–249. doi:10.1111/j.1439-0310.1979.tb00290.x.

Babson, K. A., Sottile, J. and Morabito, D. (2017) 'Cannabis, cannabinoids, and sleep: a review of the literature', Current Psychiatry Reports, 19(4), 23. doi:10.1007/s11920-017-0775-9.

Barratt, E. S., Beaver, W. and White, R. (1974) 'The effects of marijuana on human sleep patterns', Biological Psychiatry, 8(1), 47–54.

Basile, A., Hanus, L. and Mendelson, W. B. (1999) 'Characterization of the hypnotic properties of oleamide', NeuroReport, 10, 947–951.

Bolla, K. I. et al. (2010) 'Polysomnogram changes in marijuana users who report sleep disturbances during prior abstinence', Sleep Medicine, 11(9), 882–889. doi:10.1016/j.sleep.2010.02.013.

Bowles, N. P. et al. (2019) '0051 altered endogenous circadian rhythm of the endocannabinoid anandamide by body mass index', Sleep, 42(Supplement_1), A21–A22. doi:10.1093/sleep/zsz067.050.

Brooks, D. C. and Bizzi, E. (1963) 'Brain stem electrical activity during deep sleep', Archives Italiennes de Biologie, 101, 648–665.

Budney, A. J. et al. (2003) 'The time course and significance of cannabis withdrawal', Journal of Abnormal Psychology, 112(3), 393–402. doi:10.1037/0021-843X.112.3.393.

Burdick, J. A. et al. (1970) 'Heart-rate variability in sleep and wakefulness', Cardiology, 55(2), 79–83. doi:10.1159/000169270.

Calik, M. W., Radulovacki, M. and Carley, D. W. (2014) 'Intranodose ganglion injections of dronabinol attenuate serotonin-induced apnea in Sprague-Dawley rat', Respiratory Physiology and Neurobiology, 190(1), 20–24. doi:10.1016/j.resp.2013.10.001.

Carley, D. W. et al. (2002) 'Functional role for cannabinoids in respiratory stability during sleep', Sleep, 25(4), 388–395. doi:10.1093/sleep/25.4.388.

Carley, D. W. et al. (2018) 'Pharmacotherapy of apnea by cannabimimetic enhancement, the PACE clinical trial: effects of dronabinol in obstructive sleep apnea', Sleep, 41(1), zsx184. doi:10.1093/sleep/zsx184.

Chou, T. C. et al. (2003) 'Critical role of dorsomedial hypothalamic nucleus in a wide range of behavioral circadian rhythms', Journal of Neuroscience, 23(33), 10691–10702. doi:10.1523/jneurosci.23-33-10691.2003.

Coccagna, G. et al. (1971) 'Arterial pressure changes during spontaneous sleep in man', Electroencephalography and Clinical Neurophysiology, 31(3), 277–281. doi:10.1016/0013-4694(71)90098-8.

Cousens, K. and DiMascio, A. (1973) '(-)δ9 THC as an hypnotic – an experimental study of three dose levels', Psychopharmacologia, 33 (4), 355–364. doi:10.1007/BF00437513.

Cravatt, B. F. et al. (1995) 'Chemical characterization of a family of brain lipids that induce sleep', Science, 268(5216), 1506–1509. doi:10.1126/science.7770779.

Dement, W. and Kleitman, N. (1957) 'Cyclic variations in EEG during sleep and their relation to eye movements, body motility, and dreaming', Electroencephalography and Clinical Neurophysiology, 9(4), 673–690. doi:10.1016/0013-4694(57)90088-3.

Feinberg, I. et al. (1975) 'Effects of high dosage delta-9-tetrahydrocannabinol on sleep patterns in man', Clinical Pharmacology &

Therapeutics, 17(4), 458–466. doi:10.1002/cpt1975174458.

Feinberg, I. et al. (1976) 'Effects of marijuana extract and tetrahydrocannabinol on electroencephalographic sleep patterns', Clinical Pharmacology & Therapeutics, 19(6), 782–794. doi:10.1002/cpt1976196782.

Hanlon, E. C. et al. (2015) 'Circadian rhythm of circulating levels of the endocannabinoid 2 arachidonoylglycerol', Journal of Clinical Endocrinology and Metabolism, 100(1), 220–226. doi:10.1210/jc.2014-3455.

Jouvet, M. and Michel, F. (1959) '[Electromyographic correlates of sleep in the chronic decorticate and mesencephalic cat]', Comptes Rendus des Seances de la Societe de Biologie et de ses Filiales, 153(3), 422–425.

Koethe, D. et al. (2009) 'Anandamide elevation in cerebrospinal fluid in initial prodromal states of psychosis', British Journal of Psychiatry, 194(4), 371–372. doi:10.1192/bjp.bp.108.053843.

Lerner, R. A. et al. (1994) 'Cerebrodiene: a brain lipid isolated from sleep-deprived cats', Proceedings of the National Academy of Sciences of the United States of America, 91 (20), 9505–9508. doi:10.1073/pnas.91.20.9505.

Liu, C. and Reppert, S. M. (2000) 'GABA synchronizes clock cells within the suprachiasmatic circadian clock', Neuron, 25 (1), 123–128. doi:10.1016/s0896-6273(00)80876-4.

Lu, J. et al. (2000) 'Effect of lesions of the ventrolateral preoptic nucleus on NREM and REM sleep', Journal of Neuroscience, 20(10), 3830–3842. doi:10.1523/jneurosci.20-10-03830.2000.

Lu, J, Sherman, D. and Saper, C. (2006) 'A putative flip–flop switch for control of REM sleep', Nature, 441, 589–594. doi:10.1038/nature04767.

Martinez-Vargas, M. et al. (2003) 'Sleep modulates cannabinoid receptor 1 expression in the pons of rats', Neuroscience, 117(1), 197–201. doi:10.1016/S0306-4522(02)00820-5.

Martinez-Vargas, M. et al. (2013) 'Does the neuroprotective role of anandamide display diurnal variations?', *International Journal of Molecular Sciences*, 14(12), 23341–23355. doi:10.3390/ijms141223341.

McCarley, R. W. (2011) 'Neurobiology of REM sleep', *Handbook of Clinical Neurology*, 98, 151–171. doi:10.1016/B978-0-444-52006-7.00010-1.

Mendelson, W. B. *et al.* (1979) 'The regulation of insulin-induced and sleep-related human growth hormone secretion: a review', *Psychoneuroendocrinology*, 4(4), 341–349. doi:10.1016/0306-4530(79)90017-9.

Mendelson, W. B. and Basile, A. (1999) 'The hypnotic actions of oleamide are blocked by a cannabinoid receptor antagonist', *NeuroReport*, 10, 3237–3239.

Mendelson, W. B. and Basile, A. S. (2001) 'The hypnotic actions of the fatty acid amide, oleamide', *Neuropsychopharmacology*, 25(5 Suppl), S36–S39. doi:10.1016/S0893-133X(01)00341-4.

Moore, R. Y. and Lenn, N. J. (1972) 'A retinohypothalamic projection in the rat', *Journal of Comparative Neurology*, 146(1), 1–14. doi:10.1002/cne.901460102.

Murillo-Rodríguez, E. *et al.* (2001) 'Oleamide modulates memory in rats', *Neuroscience Letters*, 313(1–2), 61–64. doi:10.1016/S0304-3940(01)02256-X.

Murillo-Rodríguez, E. *et al.* (2006) 'Cannabidiol, a constituent of *Cannabis sativa*, modulates sleep in rats', *FEBS Letters*, 580(18), 4337–4345. doi:10.1016/j.febslet.2006.04.102.

Murillo-Rodriguez, E., Désarnaud, F. and Prospéro-García, O. (2006) 'Diurnal variation of arachidonoylethanolamine, palmitoylethanolamide and oleoylethanolamide in the brain of the rat', *Life Sciences*, 79(1), 30–37. doi:10.1016/j.lfs.2005.12.028.

National Academy of Sciences, Engineering, and Medicine (2017) *The Health Effects of Cannabis and Cannabinoids: The Current State of Evidence and Recommendations for Research*. Washington, DC: National Academies Press.

Navarro, L. *et al.* (2003) 'Potential role of the cannabinoid receptor CB1 in rapid eye movement sleep rebound', *Neuroscience*, 120(3), 855–859. doi:10.1016/s0306-4522(03)00339-7.

Newman, A. B. *et al.* (2005) 'Progression and regression of sleep-disordered breathing with changes in weight: The Sleep Heart Health Study', *Archives of Internal Medicine*, 165(20), 2408–2413. doi:10.1001/archinte.165.20.2408.

Nichols, K. K. *et al.* (2007) 'Identification of fatty acids and fatty acid amides in human meibomian gland secretions', *Investigative Ophthalmology and Visual Science*, 48(1), 34–39. doi:10.1167/iovs.06-0753.

Nicholson, A. N. *et al.* (2004) 'Effect of Δ-9-tetrahydrocannabinol and cannabidiol on nocturnal sleep and early-morning behavior in young adults', *Journal of Clinical Psychopharmacology*, 24(3), 305–313. doi:10.1097/01.jcp.0000125688.05091.8f.

Nishino, S. (2013) 'Neurotransmitters and neuropharmacology of sleep/wake regulations', in C. A. Kushida (ed.), *Encyclopedia of Sleep*, London: Academic Press, pp. 395–406. doi:10.1016/b978-0-12-378610-4.00087-5.

Perron, R. R., Tyson, R. L. and Sutherland, G. R. (2001) 'Δ9-Tetrahydrocannabinol increases brain temperature and inverts circadian rhythms', *NeuroReport*, 12(17), 3791–3794. doi:10.1097/00001756-200112040-00038.

Piomelli, D. *et al.* (2017) 'A Guide to the National Academy of Science Report on Cannabis: An Exclusive Discussion with Panel Members', *Cannabis and Cannabinoid Research*, 2(1), 155–159. doi:10.1089/can.2017.29009.dpi.

Pivik, R. T. *et al.* (1972) 'Delta-9-tetrahydrocannabinol and synhexl: effects on human sleep patterns', *Clinical Pharmacology & Therapeutics*, 13(3), 426–435. doi:10.1002/cpt1972133426.

Prasad, C. N. (2013) 'Obstructive sleep apnea hypopnea syndrome – Indian scenario', *Perspectives in Medical Research*, 1(1), 22–25.

Reinarman, C. *et al.* (2011) 'Who are medical marijuana patients? Population characteristics from nine California assessment clinics', *Journal of Psychoactive*

Drugs, 43(2), 128–135. doi:10.1080/02791072.2011.587700.

Rueda-Orozco, P. E. *et al.* (2010) 'Intrahippocampal administration of anandamide increases REM sleep', *Neuroscience Letters*, 473(2), 158–162. doi:10.1016/j.neulet.2010.02.044.

Sanford, A. E., Castillo, E. and Gannon, R. L. (2008) 'Cannabinoids and hamster circadian activity rhythms', *Brain Research*, 1222, 141–148. doi:10.1016/j.brainres.2008.05.048.

Schofield, D. *et al.* (2006) 'Reasons for cannabis use in psychosis', *Australian and New Zealand Journal of Psychiatry*, 40(6–7), 570–574. doi:10.1111/j.1440-1614.2006.01840.x.

Sherin, J. E. *et al.* (1996) 'Activation of ventrolateral preoptic neurons during sleep', *Science*, 271(5246), 216–219. doi:10.1126/science.271.5246.216.

Shirakawa, T. et al. (2000) 'Synchronization of circadian firing rhythms in cultured rat suprachiasmatic neurons', *European Journal of Neuroscience*, 12, 2833–2838. doi:10.1046/j.1460-9568.2000.00170.x.

Sládek, M., Houdek, P. and Sumová, A. (2019) 'Circadian profiling reveals distinct regulation of endocannabinoid system in the rat plasma, liver and adrenal glands by light-dark and feeding cycles', *Biochimica et Biophysica Acta (BBA) – Molecular and Cell Biology of Lipids*, 1864(12), 1–3. doi:10.1016/j.bbalip.2019.158533.

Stickgold, R. (2013) 'Parsing the role of sleep in memory processing', *Current Opinion in Neurobiology*, 23(5), 847–853. doi:10.1016/j.conb.2013.04.002.

Tucker, M. A. *et al.* (2006) 'A daytime nap containing solely non-REM sleep enhances declarative but not procedural memory', *Neurobiology of Learning and Memory*, 86(2), 241–247. doi:10.1016/j.nlm.2006.03.005.

Valenti, M. *et al.* (2004) 'Differential diurnal variations of anandamide and 2-arachidonoyl- glycerol levels in rat brain', *Cellular and Molecular Life Sciences*, 61, 945–950.

Vaughn, L. K. *et al.* (2010) 'Endocannabinoid signalling: has it got rhythm?', *British Journal of Pharmacology*, 160(3), 530–543. doi:10.1111/j.1476-5381.2010.00790.x.

Wong, M. M., Brower, K. J. and Zucker, R. A. (2009) 'Childhood sleep problems, early onset of substance use and behavioral problems in adolescence', *Sleep Medicine*, 10(7), 787–796. doi:10.1016/j.sleep.2008.06.015.

Cannabinoids and Inflammation and Autoimmune Disorders

Natural forces within us are the true healers of disease.

Hippocrates, Epidemics 6

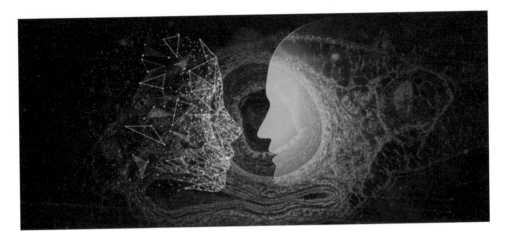

- There are no cannabinoid products approved currently for use in immunology and rheumatology diseases.
- Preclinical models of rheumatoid arthritis (RA) have reported significant antinociceptive effects related to the use of Δ^9-tetrahydrocannabinol (THC) and cannabidiol (CBD).
- The endocannabinoids N-arachidonoylethanolamide (anandamide; AEA) and 2-arachidonoylglycerol (2-AG) are present in the synovial fluid of patients with RA but are absent in normal controls.
- Cannabinoid 1 (CB_1) receptors are found in the mucosa and neuromuscular layers of the colon. Activation of this receptor in preclinical studies inhibits gastric and intestinal transit.
- In a small graft-versus-host study in patients undergoing hematopoietic transplantation, CBD appeared to show immunosuppressive properties.
- CB_2 receptor activation may modulate cannabinoid immunosuppression of inflammatory bowel disease (IBD).
- Several observational studies have reported patients with IBD that have failed standard treatments have fewer symptoms with smoked cannabis.

Introduction

The immune system is a complex system and an essential function critical for good health and survival. Cannabinoid-based treatments hold great promise for future therapeutic uses although our clinical knowledge remains very limited. In this chapter we will review selected preclinical and clinical information that may provide the clinician some insight about the future development of cannabinoids to treat immune diseases. Patients are constantly aware through the internet of numerous anecdotal reports and promotional claims about cannabinoids as remedies and appropriately ask their doctor about recommendations. In such situations the clinician should be aware that the US Food and Drug Administration (FDA), Canada Health and the European Medicines Agency (EMA) have yet to approve any cannabinoid for use in the treatment of immune-related illness.

Although a growing number of countries and multiple states in the USA have legalized marijuana for medical use by their citizens, legalization is not the same as a regulatory approval to prescribe a drug for clinical use. For approval a drug must be shown in adequately powered clinical trials to demonstrate both safety and efficacy in the treatment of a specific disease. In addition, once approved, the drug is monitored for continuing safety and efficacy and can be withdrawn from the market if concerns arise.

In Chapter 5 we briefly discussed the issues regarding the safety of cannabinoids. These concerns still remain despite the intense promotional and social pressures to use cannabinoids for medical or recreational purposes. Although the emerging data are promising and deserve further study, clinicians should always prioritize the safety of their patient before making any recommendation to use a drug where information is incomplete, including any of the cannabinoids.

In many instances approved medications fail to adequately treat the patient and the clinician may decide to prescribe a drug approved for one indication for another. This is termed off-label and is within the scope of medical practice. However, medical marijuana is not approved for any prescription and the doctor can only advise. Perhaps it is an example of the strange issues prescribers face when cannabis remains a schedule I substance but can be dispensed for recreational use in several US states and two countries.

Several professional medical societies have advised against the use of cannabinoids in the care of patients. In 2017 the National Academy of Medicine convened a committee of expert scientists and clinicians in 2017 and published *The Health Effects of Cannabis and Cannabinoids: The Current State of Evidence and Recommendations for Research* (National Academy of Sciences, Engineering, and Medicine, 2017). This was an update from an earlier report in 1999 and reviewed the medical literature published in the intervening years. Over 24,000 articles were identified and data from over 10,000 were reviewed for the report (Piomelli *et al.*, 2017).

The report concluded that there was conclusive or substantial evidence that cannabis or cannabinoids are effective for the treatment of chronic pain in adults, nausea and vomiting related to cancer chemotherapy and symptoms of spasticity associated with multiple sclerosis. The report also noted moderate evidence that cannabinoids may be beneficial in sleep disorders associated with several chronic illnesses (National Academy of Sciences, Engineering, and Medicine, 2017).

The committee recommended several areas of research to address the gaps in scientific knowledge. After the report three large, randomized clinical trials on pediatric refractory epilepsy treated with a pharmaceutical pure cannabidiol (CBD) Epidiolex were completed and led to its approval in the USA and EU for treatment of several refractory seizure disorders in children over the age of two.

We have already discussed the importance of cannabinoids in the function of the central and peripheral nervous systems in earlier chapters. Cannabinoids may be as equally critical for the proper function of the immune system. In this chapter we will review selected preclinical and clinical information regarding the relationship between the immune system and the endocannabinoid system (ECS). Preclinical studies are very suggestive of cannabinoids being important elements in both a functioning and an impaired immune system. In the future we may have medicines to address these conditions but for now no cannabinoid products have been approved for use in immune disorders.

Overview of the Immune System

In the summer of 430 BC, the Greek historian Thucydides reported in *History of the Peloponnesian War* about the plague that followed the Spartan invasion of Athens. Over one-third of the city's population were left dead from the infection. Thucydides commented he would leave speculation about the cause of the plague to others; however, he observed "Yet it was with those who had recovered from the disease that the sick and dying found most compassion. These knew what it was from experience and now had no fear for themselves; for the same man was never attacked twice – never at least fatally" (Thucydides, 430 BC).

Although resistance to acquiring infectious diseases has been recorded for centuries, the scientific understanding of the immune system dates more recently from the late-eighteenth and nineteenth century with the discoveries of Edward Jenner, Robert Koch and Louis Pasteur. Our awareness of the possible therapeutic benefits from cannabinoids is as ancient as the use of cannabis by man but our scientific knowledge has only just begun.

The innate and adaptive (sometimes referred to as acquired) immune systems are responses by the body to defend against external dangers including pathogens and internal threats. Together, these two systems provide a complex immunological defense that consists of numerous cell types and molecules including monocytes, macrophages, neutrophils, dendritic cells, cytokines, chemokines and B and T cells (Haynes, Soderberg and Fauci, 2017). Phytocannabinoids have long been known to function as immunosuppressants and recent investigations of the ECS confirm that cannabinoids interact with many of these immune cells and may potentially modulate the immune system.

The innate immune system is the older of the two defensive systems and first appeared in plants and fungi and later evolved parallel in vertebrates with the adaptive system occurring later. The first line of defense, the innate system detects an invading pathogen or other threat to the body and summons specialized white cells and phagocytes (dendritic cells and macrophages). Cytokines and chemokines, protein messengers that communicate with other cells in the immune system, are released from the macrophages and dendritic cells and the immune response is initiated. In addition to the phagocytes, other elements including complement proteins and natural killer (NK) cells are recruited in the initial response. Within a few hours, the inflammatory response is underway.

The adaptive immune system is the second layer of protection and arose after the innate system in vertebrates to provide a more targeted defense against specific threats in the environment. B lymphocytes and T lymphocytes both serve critical roles in the adaptive immune response and coordinate defenses against identified pathogens. Originating from stem cells in the bone marrow, T lymphocytes migrate to the thymus and develop into mature T helper (Th) cells or cytotoxic (T_C) cells. These T cells express CD4 or CD8 co-receptors on their surface and these protein receptors determine whether the lymphocyte will become a Th cell that activates B lymphocytes or become a T_C cell that will destroy infected cells.

In contrast, B lymphocytes remain sequestered within the marrow and manufacture B-cell receptor (BCR) proteins that coat the lymphocyte's surface and bind antigen when presented. Each B-cell lymphocyte has one unique BCR and either differentiates into plasma cells after binding to antigen or becomes a second type of cell called B memory cells. Plasma cells are B lymphocytes that have specialized into antibody factories and they begin duplication of multiple copies of antigen-specific antibodies. The release of these antibodies into the circulation is referred to as the humoral response. The second type, B memory cells, retain information on the specific antigen and are available to replicate the antibody response if future encounters occur.

Antigen-presenting cells (APC) (dendritic cells and macrophages) are specialized cells that present antigen and co-stimulatory molecules required to activate Th cells to initiate the adaptive immune system. More recently, pattern recognition receptors (referred to as Toll receptors) have been identified, especially in the skin, that detect molecules on microbial pathogens including lipopolysaccharides on gram-negative bacteria and assist the immune system to distinguish "self" from "non-self" (Sompayrac, 2012; Haynes, Soderberg and Fauci, 2017).

The opportunity to study the relationship between the immune system and cannabinoids began with the identification in the 1980s of the ECS. Our knowledge of the ECS and the immune system has continued to evolve, and the importance of this interaction likely rivals the importance of the ECS in the central nervous system (CNS). By the 1990s, the presence of cannabinoid (CB_1 and CB_2) receptors on human leukocytes was established and shortly followed by the discovery that the endocannabinoids 2-arachidonoylglycerol (2-AG) and N-arachidonoylethanolamide (anandamide; AEA) along with their synthetic and degradative pathways were abundant in the immune system.

Cannabinoids and the Immune System

The ECS has a significant presence within the immune system and serves multiple roles in activating the immune response. The CB_1 and CB_2 receptors are prominently expressed on the surface of B cells and, to a lesser degree, on other cells including NK cells, macrophages, and their monocytic precursor, neutrophils and dendritic cells (Graham et al., 2010). Activated T cells are required for the stimulation of the B-cell response although they have little or no expression of cannabinoid receptors in the resting state. After activation of the T cell by professional APCs, rapid upregulation of the receptor follows with high levels of CB_2 receptor produced (Carlisle et al., 2002). Although CB_1 receptors are the main cannabinoid targets in the CNS, it is reversed in the immune system with CB_2 receptors the most prevalent. In the peripheral immune system, the CB_2 receptor is expressed from 10 to 100 times more than CB_1 (Carlisle et al., 2002) and within the CNS, macrophages are present as microglial cells and become upregulated to express CB_2 receptors after stimulation by antigens and cytokine signaling that have intruded into the CNS. CB_1 receptors have also been found in microglial tissue and they have been reported to be present in astrocytes and oligodendrocytes (subsets of microglia) although the significance of this observation remains unknown (Molina-Holgado *et al.*, 2002).

Endocannabinoids are also synthesized in the immune cells and, as discussed earlier in Chapter 2, bind to both cannabinoid and non-cannabinoid receptors. Cabral *et al.* (1995) were the first to report that AEA inhibited macrophages from attacking tumor necrosis factor (TNF)-producing cells in alveolar tissue. Follow-up work quickly established that AEA also inhibited mouse macrophages with reduction of pro-inflammatory cytokines including the interleukins IL-6, IL-12 and IL-23 and nitric oxide (NO) (Chiurchiù, Leuti and Maccarrone, 2015). The same group also reported that AEA could induce the synthesis of IL-10, an anti-inflammatory cytokine produced primarily by macrophages and monocytes (Chiurchiù, Leuti and Maccarrone, 2015).

AEA has also been found to interact with other immune cells including dendritic cells and neutrophils. The pro-inflammatory cytokines TNFα, IL-6, IL-12 and interferon alpha (IFNα) have been found to be inhibited by AEA in dendritic cells (Chiurchiù *et al.*, 2013) and the migration and phagocytic properties of neutrophils are reduced (McHugh *et al.*, 2008, 2012). AEA is also a major immunosuppressor of the adaptive system. Through activating CB_2 receptors, AEA suppresses the release of inflammatory cytokines including IL-2- and IFNα-producing Th1 and Th17 cells (Jackson, Nagarkatti and Nagarkatti, 2014). Finally, AEA anti-proliferative effects on CD4 and CD8 T cells have been reported.

Although the anti-inflammatory effects of AEA are now well established, the same is not true of 2-AG. Inhibition of the pro-inflammatory cytokines TNFα and IL-6 and increased macrophage phagocytosis has been reported with 2-AG in the regulation of the innate system. In contrast, 2-AG has been reported to increase other pro-inflammatory chemokines and NO with an increase in cellular migration and adhesion during the inflammatory process. One report speculated that the pro-inflammatory response of 2-AG may be the result of conversion into metabolites atypical of the usual degradation of this endocannabinoid (Alhouayek and Muccioli, 2014). As discussed previously in Chapter 3, 2-AG is primarily degraded by monoacylglycerol lipase and several related hydrolyzing enzymes to arachidonic acid. However, other enzymes including cyclooxygenase 2 (COX-2) also metabolize 2-AG and produce additional lipids that are not usually associated with endocannabinoid inactivation and may be either pro- or anti-inflammatory.

Information about the role of 2-AG in the activation of the immune system is more limited. For example, there is significant suppression of IL-2, an interleukin that regulates maturation of T-cells, independent of the cannabinoid receptors. It has been proposed that this complex effect by 2-AG on the adaptive system is through binding to the peroxisome proliferator-activated receptor gamma (PPARγ) receptor and changes in gene expression (Rockwell *et al.*, 2006).

Phytocannabinoids also demonstrate significant effects on the immune system. Administration of cannabis has been found to suppress lymphocytes and macrophages (Daul and Heath, 1975; Cabral *et al.*, 1991). Δ^9-Tetrahydrocannabinol (THC) was reported to suppress the production of IL-12 and IFNγ and increase differentiation from Th cells to T_C cells through stimulation by the cytokine IL-4 (Newton, Klein and Friedman, 1994; Klein *et al.*, 2003) in infected mice spleen cells. It also appears that phytocannabinoids may have a dose effect with activation by THC at low concentrations while higher doses exhibit immunosuppressive actions (Tanasescu and Constantinescu, 2010).

CBD also appears to have immunosuppressive properties. In a nonrandomized, unblinded clinical trial of patients undergoing allogenic hematopoietic transplantation and standard immunosuppressive treatment, CBD 300 mg orally was given to patients for 7 days before surgery and for the following 30 days post-transplant. Although the study did not have a comparison group, compared with expected outcomes from other transplant procedures, the investigators reported a reduction of graft-versus-host disease (Yeshurun et al., 2015).

There are clinical situations, however, when the immunosuppressive properties of cannabinoids may be very concerning for patients with serious infection or compromised immune function. In one animal study, THC exposure in mice infected with *Candida albicans* displayed a decreased function of B-lymphocyte memory cells (Blumstein et al., 2014). Other preclinical studies have added to these concerns with reports of increased viral replication in herpes simplex virus-2, HIV-1 and several other viral infections (Reiss, 2010; Eisenstein and Meissler, 2015). In vitro studies of immune cells harvested from human donors have also reported immunosuppression by THC (Specter, Lancz and Goodfellow, 1991; Shay et al., 2003). Finally, several observational studies that reviewed long-term cannabis use reported increased rates of infection (Friedman, Klein and Specter, 1991; Klein et al., 2003; Molina et al., 2015).

Despite these preclinical and in vitro reports suggesting immunosuppressant properties of cannabinoids are especially important in immunocompromised patients, actual clinical studies do not support these conclusions. In contrast, in studies of smoked THC or oral cannabinoids, compromised patients appeared to be at no greater risk for infection (Wang et al., 2008). HIV-positive patients would be an obvious group potentially at risk for greater risk of infection in the presence of cannabis. In one acute study, HIV-positive patients treated with protease inhibitors containing highly active antiretroviral therapy were randomized to either marijuana cigarettes with 3.5% THC content, dronabinol 2.5 mg or oral placebo. No differences between the groups were found in T cells, B cells or NK cells (Bredt et al., 2002). Other long-term studies spanning several years assessed blood samples of various immune cells and also could not establish progression of HIV-positive disease (Chao et al., 2008). Other studies provide further evidence that the progression in illness in compromised patients does not occur (Abramovici, Lamour and Memmen, 2018).

As our understanding of the relationship between the immune system and cannabinoids continues to progress, new indications and treatments potentially could occur. In the remainder of this chapter we will discuss rheumatoid arthritis (RA) and inflammatory bowel disease (IBD). Although the clinical data are limited and the study size small, both are possible candidates that deserve future investigation.

Rheumatoid Arthritis (RA)

RA is a chronic, autoimmune, polyarthritic illness that attacks the synovial epithelium of the small peripheral joints, tendon sheaths and bursa. The condition is systemic, and symptoms generally manifest symmetrically on both sides of the body and in the cervical spine. In addition to inflammation of the joints, extra-articular manifestations can present including pulmonary fibrosis, osteoporosis, cardiovascular manifestations such as pericarditis, amyloidosis and scleritis of the eye.

RA is the most common inflammatory arthritis and affects women three times more than men. Often RA is associated with HLA-DR4 and, less frequently, HLA-DR1.

Rheumatoid factor (RF), an autoantibody that typically is IgM and binds to the F_c portion of the IgG antibody, is present in approximately 70% of patients. Other antibodies associated with RF include anti-citrullinated cyclic peptide antibodies (anti-CCP antibodies) and these may be present prior to the clinical symptoms of RA appearing.

Other inflammatory rheumatoid conditions occur in addition to RA. Systemic lupus erythematosus and spondylarthritis are well-known autoimmune inflammatory diseases although not all rheumatoid diseases are inflammatory. Osteoarthritis (OA), for instance, is a common arthritic condition that may have local inflammatory effects without any systemic component. Fibromyalgia, as another example, may present without any inflammatory process.

Symptoms of RA include joint stiffness and reduced movement usually worse in the morning with improvement occurring during the day. Constitutional symptoms may include fever, weight loss, night sweats, and anemia of chronic disease. Acute flares can arise in the midst of a chronic course and are characterized by increased neutrophils in the synovial fluid in the hands, wrist, knees or feet. The activated neutrophils release inflammatory cytokines including IL-6 that signal to the liver to secrete acute phase reactants that further activate the immune response.

During the acute phase, multiple proteins are released and include C-reactive protein (CRP), complement, coagulation factors, alpha-2 macroglobulin, plasminogen activator inhibitor and alpha-1 antitrypsin. In the acute phase, CRP typically will be elevated in blood and fibrinogen and immunoglobulin will coat the surface of the red blood cells and increase the erythrocyte sediment rate.

Cannabinoids and Rheumatoid Arthritis

The first controlled clinical trial of cannabinoids and RA occurred in 2006 and evaluated the effects of nabiximols, a combination of THC and CBD extracted from the cannabis plant and discussed previously in Chapter 4. The study was a multicenter, double-blind, randomized, two-arm design that compared nabiximols with placebo in 58 patients diagnosed with RA. Nabiximols was administered for five weeks in an oromucosal spray containing 2.7 mg THC and 2.5 mg CBD in each spray application. Minor amounts of other cannabinoids and other constituents of marijuana are always present in nabiximols and may have some anti-inflammatory properties as well.

Nabiximols or placebo were administered with one spray actuation 0.5 hours before bedtime with actuations then allowed to increase every two days to a maximum dose of six actuations per day. Once the patient achieved their individual maximum dose, they remained at that level for a minimum of three weeks.

Pain and joint stiffness are hallmarks of RA and in this study the primary outcome was pain on movement measured by a 0–10 numerical rating scale assessed every morning. Several secondary endpoints were also obtained including the short-form McGill Pain Questionnaire (SF-MPQ) and the 28-joint disease activity score (DAS28). Pain at rest, morning stiffness and sleep quality were also obtained from patients.

The results of the study revealed statistically significant improvements on the primary outcome of pain on movement. Statistically significant improvements on secondary measures were also found including the SF-MPQ, DAS28, pain at rest, and quality of sleep were also present (Blake et al., 2006).

A subsequent study in 32 patients with OA and 13 patients diagnosed with RA was reported a few years later (Richardson *et al.*, 2008). The authors referenced the earlier study on nabiximols and acknowledged that the function of the ECS in arthritis remained unknown. They proposed that endocannabinoids serve a function in arthralgias as an anti-inflammatory or even perhaps as an analgesic. Synovial fluid from normal controls were obtained and compared with synovial fluid from 26 patients with end-stage OA and 9 patients with end-stage RA. Synovial biopsies were also obtained from both patient groups and compared. In the RA group, one patient sample was fibrotic and could not be further evaluated, six were assessed as severe synovitis and two additional samples were described as moderate inflammation. All histological specimens were rated as abnormal with 22 of 26 scored as moderate or severe.

Inflammation was also assessed by the levels of inflammatory cytokines in the synovial fluid. Levels of IL-8, IL-1β, IL-6, IL-10, TNF and IL-12 were determined in OA and RA patients and six normal volunteers. The levels of cytokines were generally higher in RA patients compared with OA patients and normal volunteers with IL-6 statistically higher than levels collected in the OA and normal volunteer groups.

Both CB_1 and CB_2 protein and RNA were present in the synovial fluid of both patient groups in addition to the endocannabinoids AEA and 2-AG. The fatty acid amide hydrolase was also measured and present in the synovial fluid of both groups. In addition, although endocannabinoids were present in the synovial fluid of both patient groups, no detectable amounts were found in healthy volunteers (Richardson *et al.*, 2008).

Animal studies of THC and the endocannabinoid AEA have reported significant anti-nociceptive effects in animal models of RA (Smith *et al.*, 1998). Malfait *et al.* (2000) reported on rats immunized with type 2 collagen in Freund's adjuvant, an animal model for RA that activates both the humoral and cell-mediated systems and results in acute collagen-induced arthritis and chronic relapsing collagen-induced arthritis. Once the onset of inflammation was observed, CBD was given at 5 mg/kg IP (intraperitoneal). Suppression of arthritic and joint damage then followed in a dose-dependent manner. Following the oral administration of CBD 25 mg, suppression in the same study found reduction of the same symptoms for 10 days. CBD 5 mg/kg IP or 25 mg oral were reported to be the optimal dosage in a bell-shaped distribution in the preclinical model (Malfait *et al.*, 2000).

Some studies in animal and human subjects have shown that the CB_2 expression is the primary receptor that regulates the immunosuppressive effect (Malfait *et al.*, 2000). As was discussed earlier in this chapter, activation of the CB_2 receptor on immune cells suppresses the release of pro-inflammatory cytokines including TNFα and Th1 helper response.

Inflammatory Bowel Disease (IBD)

Crohn's disease and ulcerative colitis are chronic inflammatory conditions of the gastro-intestinal tract and referred to as IBD. Crohn's disease affects approximately 200–300 people per 1000 and is associated with smoking and characterized as an inflammatory disease with the highest prevalence between the ages of 15 and 35 years. It is a transmural inflammation that can skip tissue between lesions and may occur anywhere in the gastrointestinal tract from the mouth to rectum. The most common site of inflammation is the terminal ilium followed by the large bowel.

The progression of Crohn's disease frequently involves the occurrence of abscesses and fistulas that result in serious infection of adjacent tissue. Symptoms frequently include abdominal pain, diarrhea, weight loss and fever. In advanced disease, blockage of the bowel requiring urgent intervention may occur.

Ulcerative colitis is less common than Crohn's disease and presents with a bimodal prevalence between 15–25 years and 60–80 years of age with a 2% greater risk for family members. The inflammation in ulcerative colitis is more superficial than Crohn's and limited to the mucosa and submucosa layers of the colon and rectum. The illness usually occurs first in the rectum and then progresses backwards through the sigmoid and ascending colon. In a small number of patients, the entire large intestine may be involved. Ulceration of the intestinal mucosa and the submucosa layers can lead to pseudopolyps that are unaffected tissue in the midst of damaged mucosa and submucosa from the inflammatory process. Bloody diarrhea, abdominal pain, tenesmus, cramping and urgency are typical symptoms of ulcerative colitis.

In one small clinical study, markers of ECS activity were evaluated in patients with colitis. The presence of cannabinoid receptors and the associated synthetic and degradative enzymes were examined in colonic tissue. Samples were collected from untreated active patients with colitis, treated quiescent patients and normal volunteers. In active colitis patients compared with the other groups, a greater expression of the CB_2 receptor was found in addition to an increase of the biosynthetic and degradative enzymes associated with 2-AG. The authors suggested that activation of the CB_2 receptor and 2-AG may be a protective mechanism to reduce colitis-associated inflammation. (Marquéz et al., 2009).

Patients using smoked cannabis frequently report relief of symptoms of Crohn's disease and ulcerative colitis after the failure of conventional treatments. The abundant presence of cannabinoid receptors in the gastrointestinal tract and the anti-inflammatory and analgesic effects of cannabinoids have provided significant interest in the exploration of cannabinoids (especially phytocannabinoid) for use in the treatment of IBD.

Lahat et al. (2012) administered inhaled cannabis in a small, open-label study of 13 patients with well-established IBD for three months. Quality of life (QOL) was measured at two points in the study along with disease activity and change in weight. Patients smoking cannabis showed significant improvement in general health, social functioning and ability to work with reduction in physical pain and depression. The average patient weight gain was 4.3 ± 2 kg during the treatment (Lahat, Lang and Shomron, 2012).

In a second small study of 21 patients with Crohn's disease, smoked cannabis was compared with placebo in a randomized double-blind placebo design. Patients were cannabis naïve and all had failed conventional treatment. The primary outcome was disease remission measured by the Crohn's Disease Activity Index (CDAI) and was collected after eight weeks of twice a day inhalation of THC 11.5 mg or placebo. Secondary endpoints were CRP, improvement in QOL measured by the 36-item QOL short form (SF-36), and a response rate of at least 100 points change measured by the CDAI.

Those patients that smoked cannabis showed a remission rate of 45% compared with 10% of patients that smoked placebo. Remission rate was defined as a decrease of 150 points or greater on the CDAI. Although the remission rate was numerically greater, overall the THC patients' response was not statistically superior to placebo. However, 90% of the THC patients demonstrated a response to the secondary CDAI measure (CDAI change greater than 100 points) that was statistically superior to placebo. QOL measured by the SF-36 was also statistically superior compared with that of placebo in addition to reduction in pain, improvement in appetite and patient satisfaction. No overall change in CRP and other chemistry and hematology measurements were reported (Naftali and Häuser, 2014).

Several observational trials have also been conducted. These trials are studies carried out in a real-world environment and evaluate patient activity and outcomes without the limitations typically imposed in a clinical trial. These studies capture the behavior of patients and the decisions made by doctors and provide information unavailable from a clinical trial. In these studies, cannabis use has been estimated to treat symptoms of IBD of 44–51% of patients at some point in their life. Many of these patients have decided to self-medicate themselves with marijuana for the gastrointestinal symptoms after unsatisfactory response to conventional treatments (Lal *et al.*, 2011; Weiss and Friedenberg, 2015). Diarrhea, stress and sleep are common symptoms patients choose to treat with smoked cannabis. The average length of time of observation has been seven years and only a small percentage of these patients reported using THC daily. The majority reported once a month or less use of marijuana in the treatment of their IBD symptoms. Most patients administered THC through inhalation directly or through combination with tobacco or vaping. Only 1% chose oral ingestion of THC as a means of administration.

Bibliography

Abramovici, H., Lamour, S.-A. and Mammen G. (2018) *Information for Healthcare Professionals: Cannabis (marihuana, marijuana) and the cannabinoids.* Ottawa: Health Canada.

Alhouayek, M. and Muccioli, G. G. (2014) 'COX-2-derived endocannabinoid metabolites as novel inflammatory mediators', *Trends in Pharmacological Sciences*, 35(6), 284–292. doi:10.1016/j.tips.2014.03.001.

Blake, D. R. *et al.* (2006) 'Preliminary assessment of the efficacy, tolerability and safety of a cannabis-based medicine (Sativex) in the treatment of pain caused by rheumatoid arthritis', *Rheumatology*, 45(1), 50–52. doi:10.1093/rheumatology/kei183.

Blumstein, G. W. *et al.* (2014) 'Effect of delta-9-tetrahydrocannabinol on mouse resistance to systemic *Candida albicans* infection', *PLoS ONE*, 9(7), e103288. doi:10.1371/journal.pone.0103288.

Bredt, B. M. *et al.* (2002) 'Short-term effects of cannabinoids on immune phenotype and function in HIV-1-infected patients', *The Journal of Clinical Pharmacology*, 42(S1), 82S–89S. doi:10.1002/j.1552-4604.2002.tb06007.x.

Cabral, G. A. *et al.* (1991) 'Chronic marijuana smoke alters alveolar macrophage morphology and protein expression', *Pharmacology*

Biochemistry and Behavior, 40(3), 643–649. doi:10.1016/0091-3057(91)90376-D.

Cabral, G. A. *et al.* (1995) 'Anandamide inhibits macrophage-mediated killing of tumor necrosis factor-sensitive cells', *Life Sciences*, 56(23–24), 2065–2072. doi:10.1016/0024-3205(95)00190-H.

Carlisle, S. J. *et al.* (2002) 'Differential expression of the CB_2 cannabinoid receptor by rodent macrophages and macrophage-like cells in relation to cell activation', *International Immunopharmacology*, 2(1), 69–82. doi:10.1016/S1567-5769(01)00147-3.

Chao, C. *et al.* (2008) 'Recreational drug use and T lymphocyte subpopulations in HIV-uninfected and HIV-infected men', *Drug and Alcohol Dependence*, 94(1–3), 165–171. doi:10.1016/j.drugalcdep.2007.11.010.

Chiurchiù, V. *et al.* (2013) 'Distinct modulation of human myeloid and plasmacytoid dendritic cells by anandamide in multiple sclerosis', *Annals of Neurology*, 73(5), 626–636. doi:10.1002/ana.23875.

Chiurchiù, V., Leuti, A. and Maccarrone, M. (2015) 'Cannabinoid signaling and neuroinflammatory diseases: a melting pot for the regulation of brain immune responses', *Journal of Neuroimmune Pharmacology*, 10(2), 268–280. doi:10.1007/s11481-015-9584-2.

Daul, C. B. and Heath, R. G. (1975) 'The effect of chronic marihuana usage on the immunological status of rhesus monkeys', *Life Sciences*, 17(6), 875–881. doi:10.1016/0024-3205(75)90438-5.

Eisenstein, T. K. and Meissler, J. J. (2015) 'Effects of cannabinoids on T-cell function and resistance to infection', *Journal of Neuroimmune Pharmacology*, 12(2), 204–216. doi:10.1007/s11481-015-9603-3.

Friedman, H., Klein, T. and Specter, S. (1991) 'Immunosuppression by marijuana and components', in R. Ader, D. L. Felten and H. Cohen (eds.), *Psychoneuroimmunology*, 2nd ed. New York: Academic Press. pp. 931–953. doi:10.1016/b978-0-12-043780-1.50041-5.

Graham, E. S. *et al.* (2010) 'Detailed characterisation of CB2 receptor protein expression in peripheral blood immune cells from healthy human volunteers using flow cytometry', *International Journal of Immunopathology and Pharmacology*, 23(1), 25–34. doi:10.1177/039463201002300103.

Haynes, B. F., Soderberg, K. A. and Fauci, A. S. (2017) 'Introduction to the immune system', in A. S. Fauci and C. A. Langford (eds.), *Harrison's Rheumatology*, 4th ed. New York: McGraw-Hill. pp. 2–46.

Jackson, A. R., Nagarkatti, P. and Nagarkatti, M. (2014) 'Anandamide attenuates Th-17 cell-mediated delayed-type hypersensitivity response by triggering IL-10 production and consequent microRNA induction', *PLoS ONE*, 9(4), e93954. doi:10.1371/journal.pone.0093954.

Klein, T. W. *et al.* (2003) 'The cannabinoid system and immune modulation', *Journal of Leukocyte Biology*, 74(4), 486–496. doi:10.1189/jlb.0303101.

Lahat, A., Lang, A. and Shomron, B. H. (2012) 'Impact of cannabis treatment on the quality of life, weight and clinical disease activity in inflammatory bowel disease patients: a pilot prospective study', *Digestion*, 85(1), 1–8. doi:10.1159/000332079.

Lal, S. *et al.* (2011) 'Cannabis use amongst patients with inflammatory bowel disease', *European Journal of Gastroenterology and Hepatology*, 23(10), 891–896. doi:10.1097/MEG.0b013e328349bb4c.

Malfait, A. M. *et al.* (2000) 'The nonpsychoactive cannabis constituent cannabidiol is an oral anti-arthritic therapeutic in murine collagen-induced arthritis', *Proceedings of the National Academy of Sciences of the United States of America*, 97(17), 9561–9566. doi:10.1073/pnas.160105897.

Marquéz, L. *et al.* (2009) 'Ulcerative colitis induces changes on the expression of the endocannabinoid system in the human colonic tissue', *PLoS ONE*, 4(9), e6893. doi:10.1371/journal.pone.0006893.

McHugh, D. *et al.* (2008) 'Inhibition of human neutrophil chemotaxis by endogenous cannabinoids and phytocannabinoids: evidence for a site distinct from CB_1 and CB_2', *Molecular Pharmacology*, 73(2), 441–450. doi:10.1124/mol.107.041863.

McHugh, D. *et al.* (2012) 'Δ^9-Tetrahydrocannabinol and *N*-arachidonyl glycine are full agonists at GPR18 receptors and induce migration in human endometrial HEC-1B cells', *British Journal of Pharmacology*, 165(8), 2414–2424. doi:10.1111/j.1476-5381.2011.01497.x.

Molina, P. E. *et al.* (2015) 'Behavioral, metabolic, and immune consequences of chronic alcohol or cannabinoids on HIV/AIDS: studies in the non-human primate SIV model', *Journal of Neuroimmune Pharmacology*, 10(2), 217–232. doi:10.1007/s11481-015-9599-8.

Molina-Holgado, F. *et al.* (2002) 'Role of CB_1 and CB_2 receptors in the inhibitory effects of cannabinoids on lipopolysaccharide-induced nitric oxide release in astrocyte cultures', *Journal of Neuroscience Research*, 67(6), 829–836. doi:10.1002/jnr.10165.

Naftali, T. and Häuser, W. (2014) 'Cannabis induces a clinical response in patients with Crohn's disease: a prospective placebo-controlled study', *Forschende Komplementärmedizin*, 21(2), 133–134. doi:10.1159/000362829.

National Academy of Sciences, Engineering, and Medicine (2017) *The Health Effects of Cannabis and Cannabinoids: The Current State of Evidence and Recommendations for Research*. Washington, DC: National Academies Press.

Newton, C. A., Klein, T. W. and Friedman, H. (1994) 'Secondary immunity to *Legionella pneumophila* and Th1 activity are suppressed by delta-9-tetrahydrocannabinol injection', *Infection and Immunity*, 62(9), 4015–4020. doi:10.1128/iai.62.9.4015-4020.1994.

Piomelli, D. *et al.* (2017) 'A Guide to the National Academy of Science Report on Cannabis: An Exclusive Discussion with Panel Members', *Cannabis and Cannabinoid Research*, 2(1), 155–159. doi:10.1089/can.2017.29009.dpi.

Reiss, C. S. (2010) 'Cannabinoids and viral infections', *Pharmaceuticals*, 3(6), 1873–1886. doi:10.3390/ph3061873.

Richardson, D. *et al.* (2008) 'Characterisation of the cannabinoid receptor system in synovial tissue and fluid in patients with osteoarthritis and rheumatoid arthritis', *Arthritis Research and Therapy*, 10(2), 1–14. doi:10.1186/ar2401.

Rockwell, C. E. *et al.* (2006) 'Interleukin-2 suppression by 2-arachidonyl glycerol is mediated through peroxisome proliferator-activated receptor γ independently of cannabinoid receptors 1 and 2', *Molecular Pharmacology*, 70(1), 101–111. doi:10.1124/mol.105.019117.

Shay, A. H. *et al.* (2003) 'Impairment of antimicrobial activity and nitric oxide production in alveolar macrophages from smokers of marijuana and cocaine', *The Journal of Infectious Diseases*, 187(4), 700–704. doi:10.1086/368370.

Smith, F. L. *et al.* (1998) 'Characterization of Δ^9-tetrahydrocannabinol and anandamide antinociception in nonarthritic and arthritic

rats', *Pharmacology Biochemistry and Behavior*, 60(1), 183–191. doi:10.1016/S0091-3057(97)00583-2.

Sompayrac, L. (2012) 'Lecture 1: An overview', in *How the Immune System Works*, 4th ed. Chichester: John Wiley & Sons, Ltd. pp. 1–12.

Specter, S., Lancz, G. and Goodfellow, D. (1991) 'Suppression of human macrophage function in vitro by δ 9-tetrahydrocannabinol', *Journal of Leukocyte Biology*, 50(5), 423–426. doi:10.1002/jlb.50.5.423.

Tanasescu, R. and Constantinescu, C. S. (2010) 'Cannabinoids and the immune system: an overview', *Immunobiology*, 215(8), 588–597. doi:10.1016/j.imbio.2009.12.005.

Thucydides (430 BC) *History of The Peloponnesian War*. Translated by R. Crawley in 1874. Public Domain.

Wang, T. *et al.* (2008) 'Adverse effects of medical cannabinoids: a systematic review', *CMAJ*, 178(13), 1669–1678. doi:10.1503/cmaj.071178.

Weiss, A. and Friedenberg, F. (2015) 'Patterns of cannabis use in patients with inflammatory bowel disease: a population based analysis', *Drug and Alcohol Dependence*, 156, 84–89. doi:10.1016/j.drugalcdep.2015.08.035.

Yeshurun, M. *et al.* (2015) 'Cannabidiol for the prevention of graft-versus-host-disease after allogeneic hematopoietic cell transplantation: results of a phase II study', *Biology of Blood and Marrow Transplantation*, 21(10), 1770–1775. doi:10.1016/j.bbmt.2015.05.018.

Chapter 1

Cannabinoids and the Eye

The eyes like sentinel occupy the highest part of the body.
Marcus Tullius Cicero

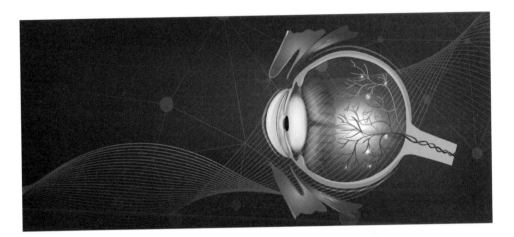

- There are no cannabinoid products approved currently for use in ophthalmology.
- Δ^9-Tetrahydrocannabinol (THC) inhaled, ingested or by intravenous administration lowers intraocular pressure (IOP). Topical application of cannabinoid receptor 1 (CB_1) agonists may lower IOP.
- CB_1 receptors are highly expressed in the human (primate) eye and are found in the anterior segment including the trabecular meshwork, Schlemm's canal and ciliary body. In addition, the choroid and retina in the posterior segment of the eye, the thalamus and the visual cortex all express abundant CB_1 receptors.
- The CB_2 receptors are located in the ciliary body, Schlemm's canal and in microglial cells in the retina.
- 2-Arachidonoylglycerol (2-AG) is more common than N-arachidonoylethanolamide (anandamide; AEA) in the normal eye, but this relationship is reversed in several eye diseases.
- Both the endocannabinoid 2-AG and the AEA congener palmitoylethanolamide (PEA) are reduced in the ciliary body and choroid in patients with glaucoma compared with those with normal eyes. AEA remains constant in the ciliary body and choroid in patients with glaucoma and in the normal eye.

- In diabetic retinopathy (DR) AEA in the retina is significantly elevated compared with the normal eye. In patients with age-related macular degeneration AEA is only slightly elevated compared with the normal eye.
- Cannabinoids have a role to play in chemical signaling of visual information, regulation of synaptic plasticity and development, and potentially neuroprotection.

In this chapter we will review selected preclinical and clinical information for future development of cannabinoids in the treatment of the eye. Cannabinoids potentially hold great promise for future therapeutic uses, but the clinical knowledge remains too limited to arrive at positive recommendations at this time. Despite the anecdotal reports and interesting findings reported over the past few decades, the US Food and Drug Administration (FDA), Canada Health and the European Medicines Agency (EMA) have yet to approve any cannabinoid for use in the treatment of eye disease.

Several professional medical societies including the American Glaucoma Society (AGS), the American Academy of Ophthalmology (AAO) and the Canadian Ophthalmological Society (COS) have all advised against the use of cannabinoids in eye disease. The AGS noted the short duration of action, side effects and the lack of evidence that cannabis use alters the course of glaucoma precluded any endorsement for use. The COS also noted the short duration of action, the possible unwanted psychotropic and systemic side effects, and the absence of scientific evidence demonstrating benefit over the course of the disease and alternative medical, laser and surgical procedures that are safer and more effective. For these reasons, the COS has not recommended cannabinoids in the treatment of eye disease.

The AAO Complementary Therapy Task Force subsequently reviewed reports by the National Eye Institute (NEI), the Institute of Medicine (IOM) and then current scientific evidence and concluded that no scientific evidence demonstrated increased benefit and/or diminished risk of marijuana use in the treatment of glaucoma compared with the pharmaceutical products already available.

In Chapter 5 we briefly discussed the many concerns regarding the safety of cannabinoids. These concerns still remain despite the intense promotional and social pressures to use cannabinoids for therapeutic or recreational purposes. Although the emerging data are promising and deserve further study, clinicians should always prioritize the safety of their patient before making any recommendation to use a drug where information is incomplete, including any of the cannabinoids.

In exceptional occasions the clinician can decide to prescribe a drug approved for one indication for another. This is termed off-label and considered within the scope of medical practice. However, on some occasions a patient is found to respond to a drug that is not approved for human use and the clinician must decide if the benefits of continued use of the medication are in the best interest of the patient. Typically, these are medications under study in clinical trials with the expectation that further scientific information will be presented and the safety and benefit of the drug will be reviewed.

The Compassionate Use Program (CUP) was passed by the US Congress in 1976 to provide seriously ill patients access to medications not approved for clinical use. Although there were no clinical trials under way to seek regulatory approval for marijuana, cannabis was the first treatment approved for compassionate use. A lawsuit was filed by a patient with severe glaucoma after he had been arrested for growing marijuana at his home and he reported that marijuana was the only drug that diminished his symptoms of glaucoma. Previous treatments, in fact, with approved medications that were available at the time had failed and the disease continued to progress. Only smoked marijuana relieved his symptoms and it appeared the only way to retain his limited eyesight was to break the law.

The patient won the lawsuit and the US government was required to supply marijuana grown at a research agricultural site at the University of Mississippi to the patient. Several years prior to this legal decision, however, Congress had decided that marijuana was unsafe for human use without any therapeutic benefit and passed, in 1970, the Controlled Substances Act (CSA) that classified marijuana as a Schedule I drug.

As a Schedule I drug, marijuana was a herb illegal to grow or possess with little expectation that scientific studies would be pursued to evaluate any potential therapeutic benefit. However, patients used marijuana for other refractory medical conditions and soon they also applied for access to the illegal herb through the CUP. Requests were approved as the potential for therapeutic benefit was repeatedly demonstrated on a case-by-case basis. To address this embarrassing situation that required the government to provide marijuana for compassionate use while simultaneously prosecuting other users, federal agencies including the National Institute of Health (NIH) and the FDA agreed to support development of a pharmaceutical substitute. With the US government conducting several of the studies and also providing funding to a small private pharmaceutical company, approval of a commercial product to replace marijuana was expedited. Dronabinol, a Δ^9-tetrahydrocannabinol (THC) chemically synthesized without any botanical ingredients, was first approved in 1985 as a cannabinoid medicine for the treatment of chemotherapy-induced nausea and vomiting (CINV) for human use.

Clinical reports had already been available for several years prior to the compassionate use approval of marijuana for glaucoma. In a brief report in 1971, Hepler and Frank (1971) first reported a reduction of intraocular pressure (IOP) in patients with glaucoma after smoking marijuana. This study was then followed up with other reports of cannabis reducing IOP in humans and animals using various preparations. Studies on smoked marijuana (Flom, Adams and Jones, 1975), intravenous THC (Cooler and Gregg, 1977) and oral ingestion all reported that THC was effective in lowering IOP (Merritt, Crawford and Alexander, 1980).

Despite these early observations and the clinical experience obtained from the compassionate use of marijuana in lowering IOP, there are no cannabinoid medications yet approved for lowering IOP in patients with glaucoma. Although dronabinol was approved for use as a prescription product, patients still preferred the illegal smoked marijuana rather than the purified approved product for the treatment of glaucoma.

Marijuana contains many other cannabinoids in addition to THC including terpenes and flavonoids whereas dronabinol is a pharmaceutically pure form of THC. The blend of ingredients in the marijuana is believed by some to produce different effects compared with THC alone. This has been termed the entourage effect and frequently is preferred by the patient (Ben-Shabat *et al.*, 1998). However, differences in formulation and the time course of absorption (inhaled versus swallowed) and the psychotropic effects make it difficult to evaluate this preference for smoked THC.

Eye drops might be a convenient way to provide cannabinoids to treat eye diseases while avoiding the issues of absorption and tolerability associated with oral dosages. Unfortunately, cannabinoids are highly lipophilic and are difficult to dissolve in aqueous solutions. Various formulations including ethanol and sesame oil have been evaluated but they are poorly tolerated and frequently irritate the eye (Green, Wynn and Bowman, 1978). Compared with currently available pharmaceutical treatment, the half-life of THC is extremely short and repeated daily dosages would be required to reduce IOP throughout the day and there would be no IOP lowering during the night.

Other studies have reported multiple effects from cannabinoids on the eye that may eventually lead to increased knowledge of the role of cannabinoids in the eye. In addition to lowering IOP, it is now well established that marijuana can reduce visual acuity, alter color sensitivity and enhance low light reception. In one report, Jamaican fishermen smoking marijuana before fishing at night were reported to have improved night vision (West, 1991). Several years later, the oral synthetic THC dronabinol was also reported to improve night vision in mountain nomads in Morocco (Russo *et al.*, 2004).

Cannabinoids and the Eye

The presence of the endocannabinoid system (ECS) has been conserved through evolution in the eye of vertebrate systems from fish to man (McPartland *et al.*, 2006). In humans, the CB_1 receptor has been identified in many locations within the eye including the conjunctival epithelium (Straiker *et al.*, 1999b; Stamer *et al.*, 2001), ciliary body and trabecular meshwork (Porcella *et al.*, 1998), nonpigmented ciliary epithelium, retinal pigment epithelium (RPE) (Wei, Wang and Wang, 2009) and retina (Porcella *et al.*, 2000). Within the retina CB_1 receptors are also abundant within the ganglion cells, cells of the inner plexiform layer, bipolar cells and photo receptors (Straiker *et al.*, 1999a, 1999b). In non-ocular areas of the visual system, the CB_1 receptor has also been found in the lateral geniculate nucleus, superior colliculus and (in the rat and mouse but not human) the suprachiasmatic nucleus (Schwitzer *et al.*, 2015). Such a diverse expression within the eye raises the question of why the CB_1 receptor and the ECS have been retained by evolution in the visual system of vertebrates.

Although the CB_2 receptor is not as extensively distributed in the eye as CB_1, it is found in several areas within the eye including the trabecular meshwork (Zhong *et al.*, 2005). Additionally, CB_2 receptors have also been reported to be colocated with CB_1 receptors and the degradative enzyme of *N*-arachidonoylethanolamide (anandamide; AEA), fatty acid amide hydrolase (FAAH), in the RPE (Wei, Wang and Wang, 2009). There is some disagreement, however, regarding the importance and function of the CB_2 receptor in the retina. Although two studies have reported the receptor within the ganglion cell layer, the inner nuclear layer and in the rods and cones (López *et al.*, 2018) numerically CB_2 has a limited presence and questionable role in retinal function.

In Chapter 3 we discussed how endocannabinoids and phytocannabinoids frequently express their pharmacological effects through receptors other than CB_1 and CB_2. The cannabinoids frequently activate these non-cannabinoid receptors and initiate processes that are not regulated through cannabinoid receptors. In addition to retinal CB_1 and CB_2 receptors, cannabinoids also bind to the transient receptor potential vanilloid type 1 receptor (TRPV1). TRPV1 is a nonselective, ligand-gated ion channel that rapidly changes the permeability of the membrane to extracellular calcium (Caterina *et al.*, 1997). The TRPV1 receptor responds to pressure in multiple areas of the body and initiates Ca^{2+} cell death. The TRPV1 channels are found in the inner retina and sense the hydrostatic pressure of IOP. In preclinical studies, activated TRPV1 channels allow the inflow of Ca^{2+} into the retinal ganglion cells (RGCs) leading to cell death and neurodegeneration (Sakamoto *et al.*, 2014).

TRPV receptors have not been identified in photoreceptors but another non-cannabinoid receptor, GPR55, has been identified on the inner segments of the rods in monkeys (Bouskila *et al.*, 2016). Previously discussed in Chapters 2 and 3, GPR55 is another G protein-coupled receptor (in the same receptor family as CB_1 and CB_2) and is nonetheless activated by the endocannabinoids, several endocannabinoid-like molecules including oleoylethanolamide and palmitoylethanolamide (PEA), and the phytocannabinoid THC. This activation by the cannabinoids originally led to GPR55 to be classified on discovery as the third cannabinoid receptor (Derocq *et al.*, 1998). However, several differences from CB_1 and CB_2 functions were subsequently reported and the classification has now changed to orphan receptor. Of interest, the phytocannabinoid cannabidiol (CBD) serves as an antagonist to GPR55 and this activity may be how CBD inhibits seizure activity rather than through the expected CB_1 and CB_2 receptors (Katona, 2015).

Endocannabinoids are also plentiful in the human eye. Both AEA and 2-AG have been identified in the anterior chamber of the eye including the cornea, iris, ciliary body and choroid (Matias *et al.*, 2006). In the retina, higher concentrations of 2-AG are present compared with AEA. This relationship is reversed, however, in patients with diabetic retinopathy (DR) and age-related macular degeneration (AMD) that have elevated retinal levels of both endocannabinoids. In contrast, patients with glaucoma have been reported to have reduced retinal levels of 2-AG without changes to AEA (Rapino *et al.*, 2017).

In multiple animal models, three degradative enzymes FAAH, monoacylglycerol lipase (MAGL) and cyclooxygenase 2 (COX-2) are also found in retinal tissue. FAAH is localized in photoreceptors, outer and inner plexiform layer, and retinal ganglion. In humans, FAAH has also been localized in the retina and especially in the RPE (Wei, Wang and Wang, 2009).

Although there are no approved therapies using cannabinoids in eye disease, the complex and extensive presence of the ECS in the visual system raises the question of why it is present and what future therapies potentially wait to be discovered. Glaucoma, DR and AMD are common causes of visual loss and blindness and the possible role of cannabinoids in these diseases remains to be discovered.

Glaucoma

Glaucoma is a chronic eye disease and a leading cause of preventable blindness worldwide. The term glaucoma is taken from the ancient Greek and refers to the blue-green haze of the cornea that can occur if the IOP gets too high. The modern-day definition, however, recognizes a broader description of the disease and describes a deterioration of the optic nerve that may eventually lead to blindness.

There are multiple risk factors that contribute to the occurrence of glaucoma with increased IOP and restriction of outflow of the aqueous humor, potentially the most common presentation. From the ciliary body aqueous humor is produced and flows into the posterior chamber around the lens and through the pupil from the anterior segment of the eye. In the posterior chamber most of the aqueous humor flows through Schlemm's canal and the trabecular meshwork sitting in the iridocorneal angle where the iris, and cornea and sclera converge. The trabecular meshwork consists of three connective tissue lamellae that filter the aqueous humor via intertrabecular channels. However, several factors can obstruct the outflow of aqueous humor and result in elevated IOP. The increase in IOP can result in neurodegenerative changes and death of the RGCs and disrupt the flow of visual information to the brain. Both Schlemm's canal and the trabecular meshwork are important in the regulation of IOP and both have abundant expression of CB_1 receptors (Chen *et al.*, 2005).

Glaucoma is a complex disease frequently (but not always) associated with increased IOP. Standard treatments for glaucoma currently focus on reduction of IOP through surgical and medical treatments although cannabinoids can also lower pressure. The extensive distribution of endocannabinoids in the eye suggests an important role for the

ECS in glaucoma that is yet to be fully understood. However, other processes also participate in the progression of the disease and can include degeneration of the RGCs and optic nerve atrophy even in the absence of elevated IOP (Rapino *et al.*, 2017).

How cannabinoids reduce IOP remains unknown although several theories have been considered. One early proposed mechanism had been that IOP is related to systemic blood pressure. In patients with systemic hypertension, however, the risk of glaucoma does not appear increased (Leske, 2002). In one study by Zhao (Zhao *et al.*, 2014), it was shown in humans that for each 10 mm Hg elevation of systemic blood pressure there was an increase of only 0.26 mm Hg of IOP. Further, in a large national study of adults using cannabis, only a modest association between recent cannabis use and systolic blood pressure was detected (Alshaarawy and Elbaz, 2016).

Smoked cannabis has also been associated with effects on the adrenergic system with drying of mucosal membranes including the mouth and in the eye. In one study in the rabbit eye, THC significantly decreased the secretion of aqueous humor along with a small increase in aqueous outflow reported through the trabecular meshwork (Green and Kim, 1976; Green, Wynn and Bowman, 1978). Intravenous administration of hexamethonium chloride, a ganglionic blocking agent, resulted in a substantial reduction of the IOP lowering effect of THC with little impact on aqueous outflow (Green and Kim, 1976).

A postmortem study in humans was conducted by Chen *et al.* (2005), and the levels of 2-AG, AEA and the AEA congener PEA were measured in cornea, iris, ciliary body, choroid and retina. Consistent with earlier reports, there was an abundance of 2-AG compared with AEA and PEA in the ciliary body, choroid and retina in normal eyes. In the postmortem eyes of patients with glaucoma, however, there was a significant *decrease* in 2-AG in the ciliary body (Chen *et al.*, 2005) when compared with the normal eye. The findings suggest that the regulation of aqueous humor may be influenced by levels of 2-AG and endocannabinoids may serve a role in the modulation of IOP.

Diabetic Retinopathy

DR is the leading cause of new blindness in the USA and Europe. Usually asymptomatic at first, DR progresses through two phases. The first phase, referred to as the non-proliferative diabetic retinopathy (NPDR), is characterized by retinal vascular abnormalities as a result of the breakdown of the blood–retina barrier. During fundoscopic examination of the eye dots and punctate hemorrhages in the retina are frequently discovered. Leakage of proteins and lipids into the retina occurs and results in cotton-wool spots and hard exudates. As vascular leakage continues, the retina becomes increasingly thicker (edema). This retinal edema may extend into the macula requiring prompt treatment to prevent loss of visual acuity. Over time, narrowing of the vessels and abnormalities of the vessels results in gradual ischemia of the retina.

The second stage of the disease is termed the proliferative diabetic retinopathy (PDR) and is characterized by neovascularization on the inner surface of the retina and progressive retinal ischemia. These new blood vessels that are formed are fragile and easily leak into surrounding tissue and vitreous; when these fragile vessels break, they result in hemorrhages. Over time the neovascularized vessels may adhere to the vitreous and retina. Traction from these fibrous attachments can result in vitreoretinal pulls and detachments of the retina, which can lead to blindness.

As the microvascular and fibrotic changes progress in DR, RGCs and cells within the inner nuclear layer can be injured or die. Even in the early stages of DR, the RGCs can be significantly reduced within the nerve fibers in the optic nerve.

There are multiple mechanisms that are involved in the progression of DR. Excitotoxicity from increased glutamate release from cells, reduced trophic factor and growth factor signaling, oxidative stress induced by hyperglycemia, and neuro-inflammation with increase of cytokines including vascular endothelial growth factor (VEGF) may all contribute to the vascular and neurodegeneration in DR (Barber, Gardner and Abcouwer, 2011). Many properties of cannabinoids potentially may contribute to these processes and influence the progression of diabetes. Obviously, more information is needed to understand the interaction of the ECS with DR.

As discussed earlier in Chapter 9, the ECS is abundantly expressed within the immune system. In the eye, the retina is an immune privileged tissue and protected from attack by both the blood–retina barrier and endogenous protective systems including the microglia and the complement system (Chen et al., 2019). The CB_1 receptor is prominent in both the retina and the brain illustrating the close relationship between the two. Similarly, the CB_2, receptor is relatively rare in the CNS and retina and is localized in microglia found in both. When threatened by a pathogen or other injurious threat, the CB_2 receptor rapidly upregulates with high expression of the CB_2 receptor expressed on the surface of the microglia (Carlisle et al., 2002). Within the microglia cells CB_1 receptors are also present in microglial tissue although their functional role is unclear (Molina-Holgado et al., 2002).

Age-Related Macular Degeneration

AMD is a progressive eye disease and a leading cause of irreversible blindness in patients over the age of 50 years (Nowak, 2006). The cause of AMD remains unknown although multiple factors likely contribute to the occurrence of the disease. Risk factors that have been identified include advancing age, white ethnicity, smoking, genetic predisposition, diet and sun exposure.

Typically, the presenting symptoms are mild and often unnoticed. Blurred vision, visual scotomas and decreased adaptation to dark requiring a brighter light to read can be the early symptoms followed by sudden or progressive expansion of central or pericentral scotomas (Jager, Mieler and Miller, 2008).

There are two subtypes of AMD that have been described and are classified as dry or geographic atrophic AMD and wet or exudative AMD. Dry AMD is the more common form of the disease occurring in 85–90% of patients with the remainder classified as having wet AMD. Although wet AMD is less common, it is usually associated with more severe visual loss.

The largest aggregation of photoreceptors (rods and cones) is found in the macula, an area that is localized in the center of the posterior retina. The macula has the highest cone density in the retina and it is the retinal area that provides us with our color perception and ability to read letters on an eye chart. Just behind the retina lies the RPE, which is one cell layer thick. These RPE cells are engaged in the phagocytosis of discarded photoreceptor segments in a process termed autophagy. Behind the RPE lies Bruch's membrane, which is a thin, semipermeable tissue that separates the RPE from the richly vascularized choroid (Jager, Mieler and Miller, 2008).

Several processes have been identified that are involved in the pathogenesis of AMD. Excessive production of drusen, neovascularization, oxidative stress associated with lipofuscinogenesis, and inflammation have all been associated with AMD (Kauppinen *et al.*, 2016).

Amorphous debris is deposited in the extracellular space between the RPE and Bruch's membrane with normal aging. This debris is termed drusen and they are subretinal deposits of lipids, lipoproteins, various cellular debris including apolipoprotein E (APOE) and oxidative and inflammatory factors (Kauppinen *et al.*, 2016). Development of drusen occurs over many years and is a complex process. In AMD, excessive deposits of drusen accumulate in the subretinal space and are classified as either "hard" or "soft" dependent upon their size and shape (Nowak, 2006). Accumulation of large deposits of drusen is harmful to the RPE cells and photoreceptors (rods and cones) and breakdown of the RPE cells lead to inflammation and eventually retinal atrophy. Large areas of the retina can become involved in this pathological process called dry AMD and in later stages of the same disease, geographic atrophy.

VEGF, an inflammatory cytokine, can be released from immune cells during this response and initiate choroidal neovascularization. This growth of new vessels in the choroid is called wet AMD or neovascular AMD and results in vessels with fragile walls that bleed into the contiguous tissue and often lead to retinal hemorrhage and sudden loss of vision.

In addition to the ischemia-related injury to the RPE cells and neovascularization, oxidative stress related to the high metabolic activity and oxygen requirements also damages cells. One of the functions of the RPE is to maintain the integrity of the photoreceptors through autophagic breakdown of apical photoreceptor segments (Nowak, 2006). This process is referred to as heterophagy and as RPE cells age and lose function, fragments and undigested metabolites are deposited in lysosomes resulting in oxidative stress and potential damage to retinal tissue.

As discussed earlier with the accumulation of drusen, local inflammation occurs after excessive amounts are deposited. Drusen contains many potentially damaging molecules that are pro-inflammatory and activate signaling systems and initiate the inflammatory response (Kauppinen *et al.*, 2016).

Preclinical work has suggested that endocannabinoids may have anti-inflammatory and neuroprotective properties (Hampson *et al.*, 1998; El-Remessy *et al.*, 2006; Kokona and Thermos, 2015; Kokona *et al.*, 2016). A postmortem study established the presence of endocannabinoids in the choroid and potentially the retina through identifying levels of 2-AG, and AEA and the AEA congener PEA in tissue. For comparison, normal cadaver eyes from donors without eye disease were compared with eyes from patients with AMD.

Significantly higher levels of AEA in AMD eyes were found in the ciliary body, choroid and cornea. However, only a numerical trend was found in the retina. There was no difference in amounts of 2-AG and PEA detected in eyes from ADM donors and normal eyes (Matias *et al.*, 2006). Although it is unknown why increased levels of AEA were present in the choroid and possibly retinal tissue, the preclinical findings of anti-inflammatory and neuroprotective properties offer important areas of future investigation.

Finally, in comparison to AMD, earlier in this chapter we discussed the increase in levels of 2-AG found in the postmortem studies of eyes from glaucoma donors. On the other hand, AEA demonstrated significant increases in levels in DR and AMD.

Bibliography

Alshaarawy, O. and Elbaz, H. A. (2016) 'Cannabis use and blood pressure levels', *Journal of Hypertension*, 34(8), 1507–1512. doi:10.1097/HJH.0000000000000990.

Barber, A. J., Gardner, T. W. and Abcouwer, S. F. (2011) 'The significance of vascular and neural apoptosis to the pathology of diabetic retinopathy', *Investigative Ophthalmology and Visual Science*, 52(2), 1156–1163. doi:10.1167/iovs.10-6293.

Ben-Shabat, S. *et al.* (1998) 'An entourage effect: inactive endogenous fatty acid glycerol esters enhance 2-arachidonoyl-glycerol cannabinoid activity', *European Journal of Pharmacology*, 353(1), 23–31. doi:10.1016/S0014-2999(98)00392-6.

Bouskila, J. *et al.* (2016) 'A comparative analysis of the endocannabinoid system in the retina of mice, tree shrews, and monkeys', *Neural Plasticity*, 2016, 3127658. doi:10.1155/2016/3127658.

Carlisle, S. J. *et al.* (2002) 'Differential expression of the CB_2 cannabinoid receptor by rodent macrophages and macrophage-like cells in relation to cell activation', *International Immunopharmacology*, 2(1), 69–82. doi:10.1016/S1567-5769(01)00147-3.

Caterina, M. J. *et al.* (1997) 'The capsaicin receptor: a heat-activated ion channel in the pain pathway', *Nature*, 389, 816–824.

Chen, J. *et al.* (2005) 'Finding of endocannabinoids in human eye tissues: implications for glaucoma', *Biochemical and Biophysical Research Communications*, 330 (4), 1062–1067. doi:10.1016/j.bbrc.2005.03.095.

Chen, M. *et al.* (2019) 'Immune regulation in the aging retina', *Progress in Retinal and Eye Research*, 69, 159–172. doi:10.1016/j.preteyeres.2018.10.003.

Cooler, P. and Gregg, J. M. (1977) 'Effect of delta-9-tetrahydrocannabinol on intraocular pressure in humans', *Southern Medical Journal*, 70(8), 951–954. doi:10.1097/00007611-197708000-00016.

Derocq, J.-M. *et al.* (1998) 'The endogenous cannabinoid anandamide is a lipid messenger activating cell growth via a cannabinoid receptor-independent pathway in hematopoietic cell lines', *FEBS Letters*, 425(3), 419–425. doi:10.1016/S0014-5793(98)00275-0.

El-Remessy, A. B. *et al.* (2006) 'Neuroprotective and blood-retinal barrier-preserving effects of cannabidiol in experimental diabetes', *American Journal of Pathology*, 168(1), 235–244. doi:10.2353/ajpath.2006.050500.

Flom, M. C., Adams, A. J. and Jones, R. T. (1975) 'Marijuana smoking and reduced pressure in human eyes: drug action or epiphenomenon?', *Investigative Ophthalmology*, 14(1), 52–55.

Green, K. and Kim, K. (1976) 'Mediation of ocular tetrahydrocannabinol effects by adrenergic nervous system', *Experimental Eye Research*, 23(4), 443–448. doi:10.1016/0014-4835(76)90173-1.

Green, K., Wynn, H. and Bowman, K. A. (1978) 'A comparison of topical cannabinoids on intraocular pressure', *Experimental Eye Research*, 27(2), 239–246. doi:10.1016/0014-4835(78)90092-1.

Hampson, A. J. *et al.* (1998) 'Cannabidiol and (-)Δ9-tetrahydrocannabinol are neuroprotective antioxidants', *Proceedings of the National Academy of Sciences of the United States of America*, 95(14), 8268–8273. doi:10.1073/pnas.95.14.8268.

Hepler, R. S. and Frank, I. R. (1971) 'Marihuana smoking and intraocular pressure', *JAMA: The Journal of the American Medical Association*, 217(10), 1392. doi:10.1001/jama.217.10.1392c.

Jager, R. D., Mieler, W. F. and Miller, J. W. (2008) 'Age-related macular degeneration', *New England Journal of Medicine*, 358(24), 2606. doi:10.1056/NEJMra0801537.

Katona, I. (2015) 'Cannabis and endocannabinoid signaling in epilepsy', *Handbook of Experimental Pharmacology*, 231, 285–316. doi:10.1007/978-3-319-20825-1_10.

Kauppinen, A. *et al.* (2016) 'Inflammation and its role in age-related macular degeneration', *Cellular and Molecular Life Sciences*, 73(9), 1765–1786. doi:10.1007/s00018-016-2147-8.

Kokona, D. *et al.* (2016) 'Endogenous and synthetic cannabinoids as therapeutics in retinal disease', *Neural Plasticity*, 2016, 8373020. doi:10.1155/2016/8373020.

Kokona, D. and Thermos, K. (2015) 'Synthetic and endogenous cannabinoids protect retinal neurons from AMPA excitotoxicity in vivo, via activation of CB_1 receptors: involvement of PI_3K/Akt and MEK/ERK signaling pathways', *Experimental Eye Research*, 136, 45–58. doi:10.1016/j.exer.2015.05.007.

Leske, M. C. (2002) 'Incident open-angle glaucoma and blood pressure', *Archives of Ophthalmology*, 120(7), 954. doi:10.1001/archopht.120.7.954.

López, A. *et al.* (2018) 'Cannabinoid CB_2 receptors in the mouse brain: Relevance for Alzheimer's disease', *Journal of Neuroinflammation*, 15(1), 158. doi:10.1186/s12974-018-1174-9.

Matias, I. *et al.* (2006) 'Changes in endocannabinoid and palmitoylethanolamide levels in eye tissues of patients with diabetic retinopathy and age-related macular degeneration', *Prostaglandins, Leukotrienes, and Essential Fatty Acids*, 75(6), 413–418. doi:10.1016/j.plefa.2006.08.002.

McPartland, J. M. *et al.* (2006) 'Evolutionary origins of the endocannabinoid system', *Gene*, 370(1–2), 64–74. doi:10.1016/j.gene.2005.11.004.

Merritt, J. C., Crawford, W. J. and Alexander, P. C. (1980) 'Effect of marihuana on intraocular and blood pressure in glaucoma', *Ophthalmology*, 87(3), 222–228. doi:10.1016/s0161-6420(80)35258-5.

Molina-Holgado, F. *et al.* (2002) 'Role of CB_1 and CB_2 receptors in the inhibitory effects of cannabinoids on lipopolysaccharide-induced nitric oxide release in astrocyte cultures', *Journal of Neuroscience Research*, 67(6), 829–836. doi:10.1002/jnr.10165.

Nowak, J. Z. (2006) 'Age-related macular degeneration (AMD): pathogenesis and therapy', *Pharmacological Reports*, 58(3), 353–363.

Porcella, A. *et al.* (1998) 'Cannabinoid receptor CB1 mRNA is highly expressed in the rat ciliary body: implications for the antiglaucoma properties of marihuana', *Molecular Brain Research*, 58(1–2), 240–245. doi:10.1016/S0169-328X(98)00105-3.

Porcella, A. *et al.* (2000) 'The human eye expresses high levels of CB1 cannabinoid receptor mRNA and protein', *European Journal of Neuroscience*, 12(3), 1123–1127. doi:10.1046/j.1460-9568.2000.01027.x.

Rapino, C. *et al.* (2017) 'Neuroprotection by (endo)cannabinoids in glaucoma and retinal neurodegenerative diseases', *Current Neuropharmacology*, 16(7), 959–970. doi:10.2174/1570159x15666170724104305.

Russo, E. B. *et al.* (2004) 'Cannabis improves night vision: a case study of dark adaptometry and scotopic sensitivity in kif smokers of the Rif mountains of northern Morocco', *Journal of Ethnopharmacology*, 93(1), 99–104. doi:10.1016/j.jep.2004.03.029.

Sakamoto, K. *et al.* (2014) 'Activation of the TRPV1 channel attenuates N-methyl-D-aspartic acid-induced neuronal injury in the rat retina', *European Journal of Pharmacology*, 733(1), 13–22. doi:10.1016/j.ejphar.2014.03.035.

Schwitzer, T. *et al.* (2015) 'The cannabinoid system and visual processing: a review on experimental findings and clinical presumptions', *European Neuropsychopharmacology*, 25(1), 100–112. doi:10.1016/j.euroneuro.2014.11.002.

Stamer, W. D. *et al.* (2001) 'Cannabinoid CB_1 receptor expression, activation and detection of endogenous ligand in trabecular meshwork and ciliary process tissues', *European Journal of Pharmacology*, 431(3), 277–286. doi:10.1016/S0014-2999(01)01438-8.

Straiker, A. *et al.* (1999a) 'Cannabinoid CB1 receptors and ligands in vertebrate retina: localization and function of an endogenous signaling system', *Proceedings of the National Academy of Sciences of the United States of America*, 96(25), 14565–14570. doi:10.1073/pnas.96.25.14565.

Straiker, A. J. *et al.* (1999b) 'Localization of cannabinoid CB_1 receptors in the human anterior eye and retina', *Investigative Ophthalmology and Visual Science*, 40(10), 2442–2448.

Wei, Y., Wang, X. and Wang, L. (2009) 'Presence and regulation of cannabinoid receptors in human retinal pigment epithelial cells', *Molecular Vision*, 15, 1243–1251.

West, M. E. (1991) 'Cannabis and night vision', *Nature*, 351, 703–704.

Zhao, D. *et al.* (2014) 'The association of blood pressure and primary open-angle glaucoma: a meta-analysis', *American Journal of Ophthalmology*, 158(3), 615.e9–627.e9. doi:10.1016/j.ajo.2014.05.029.

Zhong, L. *et al.* (2005) 'CB2 cannabinoid receptors in trabecular meshwork cells mediate JWH015-induced enhancement of aqueous humor outflow facility', *Investigative Ophthalmology and Visual Science*, 46(6), 1988–1992. doi:10.1167/iovs.04-0651.

Chapter 11

Cannabinoids and the Skin

Your hearts are mighty, your skins are whole.
William Shakespeare, The Merry Wives of Windsor

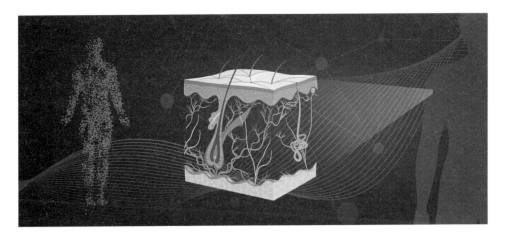

- There are no cannabinoid products approved currently for use in dermatology.
- The endocannabinoid system (ECS) is highly expressed in the skin with both cannabinoid receptors CB_1 and CB_2, the endocannabinoids *N*-arachidonoylethanolamide (anandamide; AEA) and 2-arachidonoylglycerol (2-AG), and their associated metabolic enzymes and transporters broadly distributed.
- Activation of the CB_1 receptor serves an important modulatory function in the differentiation and proliferation of keratinocytes, differentiated sebaceous gland cells and epithelial cells of hair follicles. The CB_1 receptor serves important roles both in the maintenance of the physical integrity of skin and in the immune response. Stimulation of the CB_1 receptor releases pro-inflammatory cytokines and chemokines.
- The CB_2 receptor is expressed in the basal cell keratinocyte stem cells and undifferentiated sebaceous and sweat gland cells, and in undifferentiated epithelial cells of the hair follicle. Activation of the CB_2 receptor is the trigger to initiation of the adaptive immune system.

- Both AEA and 2-AG are synthesized in keratinocytes, melanocytes and dermal fibroblasts. AEA acts as an immunosuppressant and decreases pro-inflammatory cytokines including interferon gamma and interleukin 17 from Th1 and Th17 lymphocytes.
- In addition to the classic cannabinoid receptors CB_1 and CB_2, the non-cannabinoid receptors TRPV1–4, PPARγ and GPR55 also play significant roles in the function of the ECS in skin.

In this chapter we will review selected preclinical and clinical studies for potential future development of cannabinoids in the treatment of skin diseases. Already there is a great deal of interest not only for the physiological and pharmacological properties of cannabinoids but also the potential benefits of formulations that could be provided as topical. However, this enthusiasm has not yet been matched by any regulatory agency globally and there are no approved indications from the US Food and Drug Administration (FDA), Canada Health and the European Medicines Agency (EMA) on the use of any cannabinoid in dermatology.

In the tenth century agricultural book *Geoponica*, a reference on cannabis describes the practice of applying a mixture of cannabis ashes and honey as a remedy for ulceration in the lower back (Brunner, 1977). Cannabis and honey were also used in Roman times in the treatment of wounds perhaps in part for the antimicrobial effects of cannabinoids as a treatment for *Staphylococcus aureus* (Appendino *et al.*, 2008).

The skin and its accessory structures comprise the integumentary system and protect the internal organs of the body from physical and chemical threats. The skin provides much more than a barrier, however, and is essential for the regulation of body temperature, and the sensing of environmental signals including touch, temperature and pain. In addition, the skin serves as an immunological guardian to the body and monitors the microbiota of the surface skin and the immediate environment for potential pathogens.

The accessory structures lie within the dermis and are referred to as the adnexa and are skin appendages that serve specialized functions. Sweat, sebaceous glands, eccrine and apocrine glands, hair follicles and nails are all derived from skin and comprise the skin adnexal. Among the specialized functions, the sweat glands participate in the thermoregulation of the body through secretion of water and related substances through a duct cooling the skin. Eccrine sweat glands are distributed widely on the body surface and provide the majority of cooling through evaporation. The apocrine sweat glands are generally limited to axillary and perianal areas and have minimal effects on maintaining thermoregulation in humans. The sebaceous glands produce a rich lipid sebum that reinforces the protective functions of skin through antimicrobial activity to control microbiota on the skin surface.

The skin is divided into three layers – the epidermis, dermis and hypodermis (Sams, 1990). The outermost layer of skin is a semi-impermeable boundary referred to as the epidermis. Most of the tissue in the epidermis is composed of keratinocytes and these cells begin to fill with the protein keratin as they mature and differentiate. Keratin is an intracellular fibrous protein that fortifies the keratinocyte and maintains the physical structure of the cell and protection from ultraviolet (UV) light, water loss and pathogens. Epidermal keratinocytes also express cannabinoid (CB_1 and CB_2) and non-cannabinoid (transient receptor potential [TRP] channels among others) receptors plus synthesize the endocannabinoids *N*-arachidonoylethanolamide (anandamide; AEA) and 2-arachidonoyl-glycerol (2-AG) and their related enzymes and transporters important in the function of the endocannabinoid system (ECS) in the skin (Del Río *et al.*, 2018).

The basal layer (stratum germinativum) sits on the basement membrane of the epidermis and is a single layer of undifferentiated columnar keratinocytes attached to each other by desmosomes. Basal keratinocytes are the only nucleated cells that undergo division in the epidermis, approximately every 19 days. As new germinative cells push the earlier basal keratinocytes up toward the surface, differentiating keratinocytes journey through the epidermis over a period estimated to be between 28 and 60 days. Cannabinoids serve a critical role in this migration to the surface and when disrupted may lead to hyperproliferation as in psoriasis.

Melanocytes are a second cell found in the basal cell layer and are situated freely without attachments from keratinocytes. Melanocytes serve to protect the skin from damage by UV light and contain small granules of melanin termed melanosomes. Melanocytes also contain the entire constituents of the ECS and disruption of this homeostatic regulation frequently leads to cancers of the skin.

Above the basal layer a 10 to 20 cells thick layer termed the stratum spinosum is found. Keratinocytes leave the basal layer and as they move through the stratum spinosum they begin to differentiate. The cells become polygonal in form and gradually flatten out as they are pushed toward the surface. Keratinocytes in the stratum spinosum move as single cells and frequently form and break connections with other keratinocytes. The constant activity of adhesion and fracture between cells strengthens the barrier function of skin and is influenced by expression of the ECS. As newer cells from the basal layer below push up, keratinocytes further differentiate as they move closer to the surface of the skin. Additional complex functions occur, and more keratin and glycolipids are produced. This differentiation further waterproofs the skin and protects against water loss and increases adhesion between cells.

Langerhans cells are specialized macrophages and dendritic cells found predominantly in the stratum spinosum. As immune cells, they are antigen-presenting cells and accompany antigens to regional lymph nodes and meet with naïve T-cells. In addition Langerhans cells and keratinocytes express pattern recognition receptors (PRR) that detect general classes of pathogens and together they help mount the initial immune response.

As cells mature and move through the topmost portions of the stratum spinosum, they merge into the next layer above named the stratum granulosum. Further differentiation occurs in this layer and the keratinocytes manufacture large amounts of keratin, glycolipid and lamellar keratohyalin. Together, keratin and keratohyalin give the layer a granular appearance and crosslinks form between the two proteins to give additional strength and cohesion to the cell. Finally, lamellar granules are secreted from the granular cells and coat the cell surface of the keratinocyte providing further cohesion of the physical barrier of the skin. During this period of keratinization, the cells begin to flatten out and cell organelles including mitochondria and ribosomes begin to die. Eventually the cells will become lifeless shells that contain only keratin and keratohyalin devoid of any functioning organelles.

The most superficial layer of the epidermis is the stratum corneum. Multiple layers of 10 to 30 dead keratinocytes are found and collectively provide a cellular barrier that contains keratinized cells and glycolipids closely adherent to each other. The membranes of these dead keratinized cells provide a formidable physical protection for the body from pathogens and environmental threats such as dehydration. In addition, defensins, natural polypeptide molecules produced by cells from the epidermis and the innate immune system, are found on the skin surface and serve as natural antibiotics to gram-positive and gram-negative bacteria. Gradually the adhesions between the keratinocytes are torn apart and the keratinocytes shed away to be replaced by the next generation of keratinocytes below.

In some parts of the body where thicker skin is needed for protection, another thin layer of cells termed the stratum lucidum is found below the stratum corneum. This layer consists of a border of two or three keratinocytes layered on each other and is present in areas of skin where additional thickness is desired such as the palm and soles of feet.

Below the epidermis lies the dermis. Adjacent to the epidermal basement membrane above, a thin papillary layer is present and is followed by a deeper and thicker reticular layer. In the reticular layer are found the accessory structures of skin (sebaceous, eccrine and apocrine glands, hair follicles) plus blood and lymph vessels and nerve endings.

Sebaceous glands are found in all parts of the body with the exception of the palms and soles. In general, they open onto the upper portion of hair follicle and produce a lipid rich in triglycerides and phospholipids called sebum. The purpose of this oil is to moisten the skin and provide an antimicrobial barrier to protect the skin. Elements of the ECS are prominent in sebaceous glands and disruptions can lead to excessive oiliness or dryness of the skin surface.

Eccrine glands are found throughout most of the skin and axillae and especially on the palms and soles. Located in the dermis, the gland secretes a hypotonic fluid through a duct to the surface for evaporative cooling of the skin. Apocrine glands, in comparison, are also found in axillae, anogenital, ear canal, eyelids and mammary glands region and are not involved in cooling of the body. Rather they serve as scent glands (Sams, 1990).

Hair follicles are characterized as having cycles of growth (anagen), regression (catagen) and stasis (telogen) and cannabinoid receptors are richly expressed on the surface of follicles. Cannabinoids have been associated with graying of hair and hair loss most likely associated with CB_1 receptor activation. Other elements of the ECS are also present in hair follicles and both AEA and 2-AG are produced (Telek et al., 2007). Fibroblasts are the most prominent cell in the dermis and produce collagen and the extracellular matrix elastin to provide a natural meshwork of connective tissue. Fibroblasts also produce cytokines and growth factors and contribute to the immune cells protection of the body from invasion.

Finally, below the dermis is the hypodermis considered by many not to be formally classified as part of skin. In this layer, underlying highly vascularized tissue, adipose cells and fascia covering muscle and bone attach to the skin and assist in thermoregulation and flexibility of skin. Immune cells including macrophages and lymph cells are broadly distributed in the hypodermis and reinforce the innate and adaptive immune systems in the skin in repelling invading pathogens.

The Endocannabinoid System and the Skin

Similar to the central nervous system, the ECS is extensively represented in the skin (see Table 11.1). All elements of the ECS including the endocannabinoids AEA and 2-AG, their synthetic and degradative enzymes and both CB_1 and CB_2 receptors are present. The cannabinoid system is present in epidermal keratinocytes, melanocytes, sebaceous glands and sweat gland cells, cells of the hair follicle, fibroblasts and mast cells. These cells are responsive to the influence of the ECS in normal skin function (Del Río et al., 2018; Tóth et al., 2019).

The ECS supports many of the critical functions of skin. Regulation of cell growth and differentiation, maintenance of the cellular barrier of skin, input to sensory nerve endings, inflammation and activation of the innate and adaptive immune system are all highly dependent upon a functioning and intact ECS (Bíró et al., 2009; Del Río et al., 2018; Scheau et al., 2020). The CB_1 receptor is widely expressed throughout the epidermis on keratinocytes and immortalized human keratinocytes. In normal epidermal keratinocytes, endocannabinoids are synthesized on demand to maintain the physical integrity of skin and

Table 11.1 The endocannabinoid system and the skin

Epidermis	Suprabasal keratinocytes Melanocytes	Basal keratinocytes Melanocytes	Suprabasal keratinocytes Melanocytes
Dermis	Fibroblasts Mast cells Macrophages	Fibroblasts Mast cells Endothelial cells Vascular smooth muscle	Langerhans cells
Adnexal structures	Differentiated sebaceous cells Eccrine glands and ducts Differentiated hair follicles	Undifferentiated sebaceous cells Eccrine glands and ducts Undifferentiated hair follicles Langerhans cells Mast cells	Sebaceous cells

defend against attack (Maccarrone *et al.*, 2003). Additionally, the CB_1 receptor is expressed on all mast cells and CD68+ macrophages in the epidermis and throughout the skin. The adnexal structures, as noted earlier, are present within the dermis and the CB_1 receptor is found on differentiated sebaceous gland cells and differentiated hair follicle cells. The CB_1 receptor also modulates sensory input from the skin and is expressed on large myelinated nerve fibers in the papillary dermis and nerve endings associated with hair follicles.

The CB_2 receptor is found in all layers of the epidermis and dermis as well although it is more prominent in the basal layer. Fibroblasts, CD68+ macrophages, mast cells, undifferentiated cells of the sebaceous and sweat glands and the hair follicle, and vascular endothelial and smooth muscle all express CB_2 (Del Río *et al.*, 2018; Tóth *et al.*, 2019). Within the dermis, there is an abundant expression of CB_2 receptors that modulate sensory input from small, unmyelinated nerve endings in the papillary dermis. CB2 receptors are also found on large myelinated nerve fibers in the deeper reticular layer.

The CB_1 and CB_2 receptors are both widely distributed throughout the skin and they fulfill complementary activities in maintaining healthy skin function. As noted earlier, the CB_1 receptor is present in more differentiated skin cells while the CB_2 receptor is found in undifferentiated skin cells. Together, these receptors provide complementary effects on skin tissue that regulate the differentiation and proliferation of cells (Del Río *et al.*, 2018).

In addition to the wide distribution of cannabinoid receptors in the skin, AEA and 2-AG and their associated metabolic enzymes and transport systems are also found in the epidermal and dermal layers. Keratinocytes, melanocytes, the adnexal structures and immune cells, including macrophages, synthesize on demand these chemical lipid messengers and quickly degrade them (Tóth *et al.*, 2019).

In Chapter 3 we discussed the concept that cannabinoids (both phytocannabinoids and endocannabinoids) act not only through CB_1 and CB_2 receptors but also through noncannabinoid receptors. It is hard to overestimate the importance of these non-cannabinoid receptors in the proper functioning of the ECS and this is true as well in skin. TRP channels are nonspecific, calcium channels that assist in the maintenance of the barrier functions of skin, activate sensory nerve fibers to monitor the external environment (e.g. pain, itch and heat), participate in the inflammatory process (release neuropeptides) and initiate the immune response, and help regulate thermoregulation, skin growth and differentiation (Ramot *et al.*, 2013). Similar to the cannabinoid receptors, TRP channels are found on keratinocytes, melanocytes, sebaceous gland cells and hair follicle cells, sensory nerve cells and immune cells including Langerhans cells and mast cells (Del Río *et al.*, 2018). TRPV1 is activated by AEA and 2-AG (Zygmunt *et al.*, 1999) further demonstrating the importance of non-cannabinoid receptors in the function of the ECS. In addition to endocannabinoids, phytocannabinoids also bind to TRPV1, TRPV2, TRPV3, TRPV4, TRPA1 and TRPM8 receptors (De Petrocellis *et al.*, 2012).

Another important, non-cannabinoid receptor activated by cannabinoids are the peroxisome proliferator-activated receptor gamma (PPARγ) targets. Located on the nuclear membrane, PPARγ is found in keratinocytes, melanocytes, sebaceous glands, endothelial cells, smooth muscle, and immune cells including macrophages, dendritic cells and lymphocytes. Activation of PPARγ in skin inhibits keratinocyte proliferation and inhibits the production of inflammatory mediators and cytokines (Ramot *et al.*, 2013). In Chapter 3 we discuss further the role of PPARγ and the ECS.

Selected Future Skin Uses of Cannabinoids

Although there are no cannabinoid products approved for human use in dermatology, the immunosuppressive properties of cannabinoids together with the variety of methods of delivery (oral, inhaled, topical) potentially may provide attractive opportunities to explore development of new drugs for the treatment of inflammatory skin conditions.

Cannabinoids have been associated with relief of the common complaint of pruritis. Referred to as itching, pruritis is an uncomfortable symptom that occurs as an acute (less than 6 weeks) or chronic (greater than six weeks) condition. Itching can present in many dermatological conditions including atopic dermatitis (AD), contact dermatitis, psoriasis, urticaria, infestations and xerosis among others. Multiple non-dermatological conditions can also present with itching as a symptom and include cholestasis, end-stage renal disease, multiple sclerosis, hematopoietic disease and medication side effects especially with the use of opioids (Lavery *et al.*, 2016). Although the origin and presentation can be very complex, the mechanism of action can be divided into histaminic and non-histaminic pruritus. Use of antihistamines are more effective in histaminic itch and not helpful in the non-histaminic etiology of itching.

The sensation of itch is initiated on the skin by irritants referred to as pruritogens. Pruritogens include histamine, various proteases, cytokines, neuropeptides and nerve growth factors that initiate itching by activation of long unmyelinated C fibers in the skin with cell bodies situated in the dorsal root ganglion. After decussation to the contralateral spinothalamic tract, the signal is projected to the thalamus and higher brain centers. Both histaminic and non-histaminergic circuits of itching follow separate pathways in parallel circuits to consciousness (Lavery *et al.*, 2016).

Histamine release occurs primarily from mast cells but can also occur with keratinocytes and basophils. Once histamine binds to the H_1 or H_4 receptors, the non-cannabinoid receptor TRPV1 is activated plus peptides and substance P (Yosipovitch, Rosen and Hashimoto, 2018). TRP channels have previously been discussed in Chapter 3 and are nonspecific, calcium channels that fulfill sensory (e.g. pain, itch and heat), inflammatory (release of neuropeptides) and systemic efferent functions (Ramot et al., 2013; Tóth et al., 2019)

Two small studies support the belief that this activation of the TRPV channels may occur with cannabinoids. In one study, 23 patients with end-stage renal failure and itching secondary to uremia were treated with a cream BID containing structured physiological lipids, AEA and the endocannabinoid-like molecule palmitoylethanolamide (PEA). PEA shares many of the same metabolic and transport pathways as the endocannabinoids but does not bind to cannabinoid receptors. After three weeks, 8 of 21 (38.1%) patients reported complete absence of any itching and 17 (81%) noted the absence of xerosis (Szepietowski, Szepietowski and Reich, 2005).

A second study of 22 patients with pruritis, prurigo and lichen simplex were treated only with the 'endocannabinoid-like' PEA administered as a cream. The vast majority of the patients reported reduction of itch by 86.4% (Ständer, Reinhardt and Luger, 2006).

AD is a chronic, relapsing, pruritic dermatitis that involves the breakdown of the stratum corneum and entry of pathogens into the body (Clark, Nicol and Adinoff, 1990). It presents in acute, subacute and chronic conditions and affects different parts of the skin from infants to adults. No matter how AD presents, however, pruritis is a frequent complaint and caused the greatest discomfort.

In an eight-week, randomized, single-blinded controlled study of 20 patients with AD, treatment with 30 mg of hempseed oil QID was compared with 30 ml of olive oil QID in reducing symptoms of AD. Patients treated with hempseed oil (hempseed oil is made from seeds that contain little or no Δ^9-tetrahydrocannabinol (THC) and is rich in fatty acids) were found to have significant improvement in pruritis and xerosis compared with olive oil, and to have an increase in the level of essential fatty acids measured in blood (Callaway et al., 2005).

Acne vulgaris is a common skin disease with multiple etiologies that frequently presents with itching. Noninflammatory and inflammatory acne are two common forms that present to the clinician. The noninflammatory lesions are open comedones (blackheads) and closed comedones (whiteheads). Inflammatory lesions presenting as cysts, nodules and pustules describe the inflammatory presentation of acne. Excessive secretion from the sebaceous gland or blockage of the duct are likely causes of acne. Once the secretory duct is blocked and keratinization of the hair follicle epithelium occurs, secondary infection from bacteria, especially Cutibacterium acnes (Propionibacterium acnes), initiates an inflammatory response (White, 1990).

In one recent clinical trial, cannabis seed oil (a common ingredient of lipid-based creams used for the cosmetic treatment of acne) was evaluated in a split face study. Eleven healthy adult subjects with acne or seborrheic dermatitis were treated with 3% cannabis seed extract applied as a cream to the cheek on one side of the face and vehicle only on the other. Compared with the side with vehicle only, the treated side showed a significant decrease of erythema and skin sebum (Ali and Akhtar, 2015).

As discussed earlier in this chapter, CB_1 receptors are found on differentiated sebocytes and CB_2 on undifferentiated cells (Ständer, Reinhardt and Luger, 2006). It is likely that the CB_2 receptor provides some homeostasis for the maintenance of the sebum lipogenesis. Blocking cannabinoid receptor activity leads to decreased lipid production and exposure to endocannabinoids leads to excessive production of sebum (Tóth et al., 2019). Sebum contributes to the softening of skin and provides elasticity to the barrier while also creating an antibacterial barrier on the surface and controlling the microbiological flora (Pappas *et al.*, 2009; Shi *et al.*, 2015). Thus, disruption of this control of sebum production or flow to the skin can result in dryness in AD or inflammation in acne and seborrhea (Pappas *et al.*, 2009).

Along with the CB_2 receptors, non-cannabinoid receptors are also involved in regulating lipogenesis. Activation of TRPV1–4 was shown to decrease the production of sebum (Szántó *et al.*, 2019; Tóth *et al.*, 2019) and, in the case of TRPV3 activation, release significant pro-inflammatory cytokines.

There is some limited evidence that cannabinoids may have therapeutic benefit in other inflammatory skin diseases including psoriasis, AD and contact allergic dermatitis. The anti-proliferative properties of cannabinoids plus the anti-inflammatory effects suggests the ECS may serve an important role in the pathogenesis of psoriasis. Several phytocannabinoids including THC, CBD, cannabinol and cannabigerol have been reported to inhibit hyperproliferation of human keratinocytes in vitro (Wilkinson and Williamson, 2007). In addition, cannabinoids suppress inflammation through several mechanisms (Klein and Cabral, 2006). Although the anti-inflammatory response in the disease is not fully understood, various immune cells plus disruption in lymphocyte Th1 and Th17 cells are closely involved in the expression of psoriasis (Krueger and Bowcock, 2005; Ogawa *et al.*, 2018).

Allergic contact dermatitis is an immunological response of the skin as a result of exposure to an allergen. Common causes of allergic dermatitis include poison ivy/oak, nickel, rubber compounds, paraphenylenediamine, neomycin, ethylenediamine, preservatives in topical medications and cosmetics (Martini and Marks, 1990). Anti-inflammatory effects of cannabinoids are mediated through activation of the cannabinoid receptors and are likely involved in reducing allergic contact dermatitis. In one study using a murine model to induce allergic contact dermatitis with the application of 2,4-dinitro-1-fluorobenzene (DNFB), a topical application of THC was applied as an agonist to both the CB_1 and CB_2 receptors. THC was found to reduce inflammation in the mouse skin. Using DNFB in genetic strains of mice deficient in CB_1 and CB_2 receptors or in mice treated with cannabinoid receptor antagonists resulted in enhanced contact allergic inflammation.

Because the application of THC suppressed inflammation through activation of the cannabinoid receptors, mice deficient in fatty acid amide hydrolase (FAAH) and subsequently elevated AEA levels were studied. After applying DNFB to the FAAH-deficient mice an attenuated allergic response was noted demonstrating that endocannabinoids bind to the cannabinoid receptors and reduce the contact hypersensitivity response (Karsak *et al.*, 2007).

As discussed earlier, endocannabinoids and phytocannabinoids also bind to non-cannabinoid receptors. Subsequent work followed using the DNFB murine model of allergic contact dermatitis to determine if non-cannabinoid receptors might also contribute to the reduction in inflammation. The results showed that THC inhibited the release of interferon gamma from both T cells and keratinocytes and decreased the production of several pro-inflammatory chemokines. The authors concluded that THC reduced inflammation through inhibition of keratinocyte release of chemokines independent of the CB_1 and CB_2 receptors (Gaffal *et al.*, 2013).

Psoriasis is a chronic inflammatory skin disease of autoimmune origin presenting with well-demarcated erythematous, scaly plaques that frequently itch. It appears on the epidermis extensor surface of elbows, knees, lumbar and scalp and other areas of the body including muscular and skeletal sites may be involved. Hyperproliferation of poorly differentiated keratinocytes, hypervascularity of the underlying dermis and signs of excessive inflammation characterize the disease (Norooznezhad and Norooznezhad, 2017).

In addition to changes in the skin, psoriasis is also associated with systemic changes including an increase in circulating leukocytes (especially granulocytes) and higher levels of cytokines in the blood. There are several types of psoriasis with psoriasis vulgaris and psoriatic arthritis being two of the most common encountered clinically.

Psoriatic arthritis appears to have a strong genetic disposition and presents with overlapping symptoms similar to ankylosing spondylitis and Reiter's disease. Increased severity of psoriasis and inflammation often results in greater impairment of the patient and the presence of arthritic pain (Zanolli, 1990).

Presentation of antigen to T cells and activation of B cells and initiation of the adaptive immune system is a feature of autoimmune disease and psoriasis. As discussed in Chapter 9, CB_2 receptors are present in low quantities on the T cell but in the presence of antigen-presenting cells rapidly upregulate and the immune response accelerates.

A recent study evaluated the role of the ECS in psoriasis and blood samples were obtained from 136 subjects. In the study, blood samples were collected from 68 patients with a diagnosis of psoriasis vulgaris and 34 patients with a diagnosis of psoriatic arthritis, and compared with those taken from 34 healthy controls.

Compared with the normal controls, both patient groups had higher levels of endocannabinoids (AEA and 2-AG) in plasma. Both patient groups also had higher levels of the ECS degradative enzymes FAAH and monoacylglycerol lipase in circulating granulocytes compared with normal controls. However, there were differences in expression of cannabinoid receptors between the patient groups with CB_1 higher in patients diagnosed with psoriatic arthritis and CB_2 higher in patients diagnosed with psoriasis vulgaris. In contrast, expression of GPR55, originally considered a third cannabinoid receptor and blocked by CBD (Ryberg et al., 2009), was found to be the same in both patient groups (Ambrożewicz et al., 2018). The authors postulated that the overexpression of endocannabinoids might be in response to limiting the progression of psoriasis.

Bibliography

Ali, A. and Akhtar, N. (2015) 'The safety and efficacy of 3% Cannabis seeds extract cream for reduction of human cheek skin sebum and erythema content', *Pakistan Journal of Pharmaceutical Sciences*, 28(4), 1389–1395.

Ambrożewicz, E. et al. (2018) 'Pathophysiological alterations of redox signaling and endocannabinoid system in granulocytes and plasma of psoriatic patients', *Cells*, 7(10), 159. doi:10.3390/cells7100159.

Appendino, G. et al. (2008) 'Antibacterial cannabinoids from *Cannabis sativa*: a structure-activity study', *Journal of Natural Products*, 71(8), 1427–1430. doi:10.1021/np8002673.

Bíró, T. et al. (2009) 'Novel perspectives and therapeutic opportunities', *Trends in Pharmacological Sciences*, 30(8), 411–420. doi:10.1016/j.tips.2009.05.004.The.

Brunner, T. F. (1977) 'Marijuana in ancient Greece and Rome? The literary evidence', *Journal of Psychoactive Drugs*, 9(3), 221–225. doi:10.1080/02791072.1977.10472052.

Callaway, J. et al. (2005) 'Efficacy of dietary hempseed oil in patients with atopic dermatitis', *Journal of Dermatological Treatment*, 16(2), 87–94. doi:10.1080/09546630510035832.

Clark, R. A. F., Nicol, N. and Adinoff, A. D. (1990) 'Atopic dermatitis', in W. M. Sams and P. J. Lynch (eds.), *Principles and Practice of Dermatology*. New York: Churchill Livingstone. pp. 365–380.

De Petrocellis, L. *et al.* (2012) 'Cannabinoid actions at TRPV channels: effects on TRPV3 and TRPV4 and their potential relevance to gastrointestinal inflammation', *Acta Physiologica*, 204(2), 255–266. doi:10.1111/j.1748-1716.2011.02338.x.

Del Río, C. *et al.* (2018) 'The endocannabinoid system of the skin. A potential approach for the treatment of skin disorders', *Biochemical Pharmacology*, 122–133. doi:10.1016/j.bcp.2018.08.022.

Gaffal, E. *et al.* (2013) 'Cannabinoid 1 receptors in keratinocytes modulate proinflammatory chemokine secretion and attenuate contact allergic inflammation', *The Journal of Immunology*, 190(10), 4929–4936. doi:10.4049/jimmunol.1201777.

Karsak, M. *et al.* (2007) 'Attenuation of allergic contact dermatitis through the endocannabinoid system', *Science*, 316 (5830), 1494–1497. doi:10.1126/science.1142265.

Klein, T. W. and Cabral, G. A. (2006) 'Cannabinoid-induced immune suppression and modulation of antigen-presenting cells', *Journal of Neuroimmune Pharmacology*, 1(1), 50–64. doi:10.1007/s11481-005-9007-x.

Krueger, J. G. and Bowcock, A. (2005) 'Psoriasis pathophysiology: current concepts of pathogenesis', *Annals of the Rheumatic Diseases*, 64(Suppl 2), ii30–ii36. doi:10.1136/ard.2004.031120.

Lavery, M. J. *et al.* (2016) 'Pruritus: an overview. What drives people to scratch an itch?', *Ulster Medical Journal*, 85(3), 167–173.

Maccarone, M. *et al.* (2003) 'The endocannabinoid system in human keratinocytes: evidence that anandamide inhibits epidermal differentiation through CB1 receptor-dependent inhibition of protein kinase C, activation protein-1, and transglutaminase', *Journal of Biological Chemistry*, 278(36), 33896–33903.

Martini, M. C. and Marks, J. G. (1990) 'Contact dermatitis and contact urticaria', in W. M. Sams and P. J. Lynch (eds.), *Principles and Practice of Dermatology*. New York: Churchill Livingstone. pp. 389–402.

Norooznezhad, A. H. and Norooznezhad, F. (2017) 'Cannabinoids: possible agents for treatment of psoriasis via suppression of angiogenesis and inflammation', *Medical Hypotheses*, 99, 15–18. doi:10.1016/j.mehy.2016.12.003.

Ogawa, E. *et al.* (2018) 'Pathogenesis of psoriasis and development of treatment', *The Journal of Dermatology*, 45(3), 264–272. doi:10.1111/1346-8138.14139.

Pappas, A. *et al.* (2009) 'Sebum analysis of individuals with and without acne', *Dermato-Endocrinology*, 1(3), 157–161. doi:10.4161/derm.1.3.8473.

Ramot, Y. *et al.* (2013) 'A novel control of human keratin expression: cannabinoid receptor 1-mediated signaling down-regulates the expression of keratins K6 and K16 in human keratinocytes in vitro and in situ', *PeerJ*, 1, e40. doi:10.7717/peerj.40.

Ryberg, E. *et al.* (2009) 'The orphan receptor GPR55 is a novel cannabinoid receptor', *British Journal of Pharmacology*, 152(7), 1092–1101. doi:10.1038/sj.bjp.0707460.

Sams, W. M. (1990) 'Structure and function of skin', in W. M. Sams and P. J. Lynch (eds.), *Principles and Practice of Dermatology*. New York: Churchill Livingstone. pp. 3–14.

Scheau, C. *et al.* (2020) 'Cannabinoids in the pathophysiology of skin inflammation', *Molecules*, 25(3), 652. doi:10.3390/molecules25030652.

Shi, V. Y. *et al.* (2015) 'Role of sebaceous glands in inflammatory dermatoses', *Journal of the American Academy of Dermatology*, 73(5), 856–863. doi:10.1016/j.jaad.2015.08.015.

Ständer, S., Reinhardt, H. W. and Luger, T. A. (2006) 'Topische cannabinoidagonisten. Eine effektive, neue möglichkeit zur behandlung von chronischem pruritus', *Der Hautarzt*, 57 (9), 801–807. doi:10.1007/s00105-006-1180-1.

Szántó, M. *et al.* (2019) 'Activation of TRPV3 inhibits lipogenesis and stimulates production of inflammatory mediators in human sebocytes—a putative contributor to dry skin dermatoses', *Journal of Investigative Dermatology*, 139(1), 250–253. doi:10.1016/j.jid.2018.07.015.

Szepietowski, J. C., Szepietowski, T. and Reich, A. (2005) 'Efficacy and tolerance of the cream containing structured physiological lipids with endocannabinoids in the treatment of uremic pruritus: a preliminary study', *Acta Dermatovenerologica Croatica*, 13(2), 97–103.

Telek, A. *et al.* (2007) 'Inhibition of human hair follicle growth by endo- and exocannabinoids', *FASEB Journal*, 21(13), 3534–3541. doi:10.1096/fj.06-7689com.

Tóth, K. F. *et al.* (2019) 'Cannabinoid signaling in the skin: therapeutic potential of the "c(ut) annabinoid" system', *Molecules*, 24(5), 1–56. doi:10.3390/molecules24050918.

White, P. A. (1990) 'Eczematous reaction patterns', in W. M. Sams and P. J. Lynch (eds.), *Principles and Practice of Dermatology*. New York: Churchill Livingstone. pp. 381–388.

Wilkinson, J. D. and Williamson, E. M. (2007) 'Cannabinoids inhibit human keratinocyte proliferation through a non-CB1/CB2 mechanism and have a potential therapeutic value in the treatment of psoriasis', *Journal of Dermatological Science*, 45(2), 87–92. doi:10.1016/j.jdermsci.2006.10.009.

Yosipovitch, G., Rosen, J. D. and Hashimoto, T. (2018) 'Itch: From mechanism to (novel) therapeutic approaches', *Journal of Allergy and Clinical Immunology*, 142(5), 1375–1390. doi:10.1016/j.jaci.2018.09.005.

Zanolli, M. D. (1990) 'Psoriasis and Reiter's disease', in W. M. Sams and P. J. Lynch (eds.), *Principles and Practice of Dermatology*. New York: Churchill Livingstone. pp. 307–324.

Zygmunt, P. M. *et al.* (1999) 'Vanilloid receptors on sensory nerves mediate the vasodilator action of anandamide', *Nature*, 74(9), 452–457. doi:10.1038/22761.

Index